SILVER DENTAL FILLINGS

CAN THE MERCURY IN YOUR DENTAL FILLINGS POISON YOU?

SAM ZIFF

AURORA PRESS

205 Third Avenue   2A   New York, N.Y. 10003

First published in 1984 by
Aurora Press
205 3rd Ave. 2A
New York, New York 10003

ISBN: 0-943358-22-1
Library of Congress Catalogue Card No:
84-072253

DEDICATION

To my wife Helen who supported me so unselfishly during the researching and writing of this book and whose primary reward was to become a temporary "mercury widow." To my son Michael whose intense interest in the subject convinced me to assist him in doing research on the potential toxicity of mercury and dental amalgam and to his wife Peggy who so ably assisted in editing the final manuscript.

To that small group of dentists, other health care providers and researchers who in the face of overwhelming peer and establishment pressures continued their individual efforts to prove the potential toxicity of dental amalgam fillings. Their motivating force has always been the health and well being of the patient.

Most of all this book is dedicated to the millions of people who are unaware that their "Silver Dental Fillings" actually contain more mercury than silver and that the mercury escaping from their silver fillings has the potential of seriously affecting their health.

TABLE OF CONTENTS

Foreword By Joel M. Berger D.D.S i
Foreword By Jeffrey Bland PHD iv
INTRODUCTION v
Chapter 1: MERCURY IN MEDICINE
             AND DENTISTRY 2
     Section I. History of Mercury in Medicine 2
     Section II. History of Mercury in Dentistry 8

Chapter 2: WHERE ARE WE NOW? 15

Chapter 3: WHAT IS MERCURY? 21

Chapter 4: THE ARGUMENTS FOR
             AND AGAINST 27
     Argument 1. 29
         The American Dental Association is constantly
         studying and evaluating the safety and tolerance of
         mercury used in dental restorations
     Argument 2. 30
         Dentistry need only concern itself with the potential
         toxicity of mercury vapor
     Argument 3. 33
         Recent test indicating the release of mercury vapor
         from dental amalgams in teeth may not be valid
     Argument 4. 37
         There is no scientific evidence to indicate that
         inhaling very small doses of mercury increase the
         incidence of disease or cause higher mortality rates in
         anyone including dental personnel who have a much
         greater exposure
     Argument 5. 41
         Measurement of mercury content of the urine is a
         reliable indicator of whether an individual may suffer
         any biological effects from exposure to mercury
     Argument 6. 46
         Only individuals sensitive to mercury should consider
         replacing their amalgam fillings

Argument 7. 52
    Once mercury is combined with other metals used in
    dental amalgam its toxic properties are made
    harmless
    References for the arguments 60

Chapter 5: DO WE REALLY HAVE
            ELECTRICITY IN OUR MOUTHS? 65

Chapter 6: MERCURY IN MY BODY?
            WHERE DOES IT GO?
            HOW LONG DOES IT STAY? 71
Section I. Mercury in my body? 72
Section II. Where does it go? 74
Section III. How long does it stay? 78

Chapter 7: PATHOLOGY OR DOES MERCURY
            CAUSE ANY CHANGES
            IN OUR TISSUES AND ORGANS? 83
Section I. Central nervous system (CNS)/brain 84
Section II. Renal Function 88
Section III. Cardiovascular 89
Section IV. Endocrine system 92
Section V. The Immune system 96
Section VI. Oral cavity 102
Section VII. Mercury toxicity in the human 104
reproductive cycle. Mother? Embryo?
Fetus? Infant?
Section VIII. Fantasy Land? Or real psychiatric 107
and behavioral manifestations
References. 110

Chapter 8: MICROMERCURIALISM AND SIGNS
            AND SYMPTOMS MERCURY
            CAN PRODUCE 119

Chapter 9: ANECDOTES 127

Chapter 10: WHAT CAN I DO? 143

FOREWORD
By Jeffrey Bland, Ph.D.

The field of dental amalgam and its relationship to chronic mercurial immunosuppressive disorders has recently been revived and has received considerable attention. For years it has been assumed that once amalgam restorative work is in place it becomes fixed and does not liberate mercury to systemic circulation. However, recent information seems to indicate that there are a number of variables which may contribute to increased ablation of mercury amalgams, including galvanic currents, plaque and pH of the oral cavity. Given these observations there is concern that in individuals who undergo more rapid amalgam ablation there may be enhanced accumulation of systemic mercury which could have significant influences upon the immune system through lymphocyte inactivity or alteration of T/suppressor/helper ratios. The recent work of Eggleston seems to indicate that there is a relationship between immunosuppressive effects and mercury amalgams in some patients. Given this, the book "Silver Dental Fillings: The Toxic Time Bomb" comes at a very appropriate time. It alerts the reader to the need for more research and understanding of the role that mercury amalgam may have on chronic health dysfunction. It appears that the position of many dental researchers has been that mercury is safe in the mouth as applied and does not require extensive additional research. This book seems to open the question for reevaluation and exploration and it appears that, at least for those who are mercury-sensitive and who have more rapid ablation of mercury amalgams, this message may have considerable importance in terms of their long-term health. I believe this book is going to contribute to an enlightenment in the general field and to more extensive research which is needed to compare the safety of amalgam restorative work to other alternatives such as precious metals and plastics.

Jeffrey Bland, Ph.D.
Director
Laboratory for Nutritional
Supplement Analysis
Linus Pauling Institute of
Science and Medicine

FOREWORD
By Joel M. Berger D.D.S.

There is a growing collection of scientific research indicating that mercury in dental amalgams migrates into the body and affects the immune system. Old myths masquerading as facts, die hard. The idea that the silver-mercury mixture in your mouth is stable or safe, is as true as Easter bunnies lay Easter eggs!

When the facts presented to you in this book, are fully implemented by the dental professions, they will finally be able to enter the onrushing twenty-first century, having fully missed the twentieth century by continuing to fill teeth with a nineteenth century unstable poisonous mixture.

Technology has caught up with this big lie. It is a simple procedure today for a dentist to have you chew gum for three to five minutes and then test your mouth for the presence of mercury vapor, with the Jerome Mercury Vapor Analyzer, Model 411 A. The simple demonstration of mercury vapor in the mouth, and in the air surrounding the dentist and patient during amalgam removal, surely indicates a large volume of free mercury in an amalgam.

There is no such thing as a stable amalgam filling. Each one will leak mercury in every direction: into the body of the tooth, into the gum tissue surrounding the tooth and bone, into the air of the mouth, where it is carried to the nose and brain, and into saliva where it is both carried as mercury into the bloodstream, methylated by normal body bacteria into the dangerous poison methy-mercury. We are dealing with a known and proven poison. The mercury leaking out, sets the potential for lowering the body's immune response and as a result undermining our total health. Dentists have turned people's mouths into storage batteries. Into a solution (your saliva) which is slightly acid and slightly salty, they've added metals. These metals will interact causing the measurable loss of the weakest metal, mercury and the generation of electricity. The mercury travels throughout the body, and the currents generated can locally initiate nerve impulses, affect electrical transmission from the brain to the heart and alter the many acupuncture meridians that pass through the face. This means that a problem or impulse beginning in a tooth can affect a distant muscle or organ system.

Based upon the current documented scientific knowledge and research, a dentist cannot, with impunity, introduce a metal into a patient's mouth and expect there to be no biological effect. Numerous documented studies show that the introduction of silver-mercury amalgam filling will cause leakage of mercury into the body. The later use of gold or palladium alloy elsewhere in the mouth will cause the more rapid release of mercury.

The ideal dental restoration should be:
1. As few different metals as possible
2. As little metal as possible
3. As noble as possible (gold, platinum, etc.)
4. Covered with porcelain to reduce chemical and electrical interaction with the oral environment.

An important piece of research was done by Dr. David W. Eggleston, reported in the *Journal of Prosthetic Dentistry*, Vol. 51 No. 5 P. 617–623, May 1984.

Dr. Eggleston measured the T-lymphocyte precent of the total lymphocyte count in his patients before and after the insertion and removal of dental amalgam and nickle-base alloys. The ability of dental amalgam to modify immune homeostasis is evident in this study that produced dramatic changes in the patients who participated in it. For example: in one patient, removing six amalgam restorations increased the T-lymphocyte percentage from 47% (before removal) to 73% (after removal), an increase of 55.3%. Reinsertion of only four new amalgam restorations decreased the T-lymphocyte percentage, down to 55%. Dr. Eggleston concludes "preliminary data suggests that dental amalgam and dental nickle alloys can adversely affect the quantity of T-lymphocytes." Human T-lymphocytes can recognize specific antigens, execute effector functions and regulate the type and intensity of virtually all cellular and humoral immune responses. Normal immune function depends on a proper quantity, quality and ratio of T-lymphocyte helper and suppresor subsets." Dr. Eggleston's researches have continued and he will soon publish a report on a large number of patients.

As a full time practicing dentist who is concerned first with the overall health and well being of my patients, and only secondarily with the fine art of dental sculpturing and tooth carpentry, I am able to help many of my patients improve their health by removing their mercury and nickle containing dentistry. I and many other dentists all over the world, are now aware of this serious health hazard, and are routinely removing silver-mercury amalgams, at the request of many doctors.

Mercury should be taken out of dentistry and gotten out of the human body. It does not belong there.

Sam Ziff's efforts to present this serious issue to a wider public fills a void, and it is hoped that this book will stimulate more research and a "clean up" of this "toxic timebomb" from future generations.

Joel M. Berger
September 15, 1984 Bayside, N.Y.

Joel M. Berger is a full-time practicing dentist in Bayside, N.Y., for the last 24 years, and N.Y.U. graduate, a member of both the American Dental Association and the N.Y. Holistic Dental Association. He is a well known lecturer to profesional dental organizations and frequently appears on radio and television in an attempt to bring the dangers of silver-mercury amalgam toxicity, to public consciousness.

INTRODUCTION

The greatest health controversy of our time is brewing. The issue of this controversy is whether the human body accommodates, without lasting ill effects, to its exposure to the metal mercury. Mercury is utilized in the practice of dentistry, medicine, manufacture of pharmaceutical and cosmetic preparations, industry, in agricultural applications as fungicides/pesticides, and the environmental contamination resulting from some of the applications mentioned. The final insult to our bodies being the actual consumption of mercury that has become a part of the food chain.

If our bodies do not accommodate adequately, does this mean that our exposures to mercury and other toxic metals may in fact be causing untold damage that in some instances may even be irreparable? Can it be possible that mercury may be the "key", the single factor responsible for so many unexplainable health problems experienced by man, which are of unknown origin or etiology?

It is not my intent in writing this book to address all the possible sources of mercury contamination of the human body. This book will address only its use in dentistry, which I consider to be the central issue to the overall problem of human exposure.

Simply stated, the issue is whether the standard filling material utilized by the dental profession world-wide since its invention in the year 1819 is safe.

The material in question is called amalgam and takes several forms or compositions. It is most commonly referred to as silver amalgam or just silver. The material is provided to the dentist as two separate entities which he or his staff must then mix together. The final product is then placed into the tooth cavity to fill or reconstruct the tooth. The first entity of amalgam is an alloy or mixture of the following metals: not less than 65% silver; not less than 25% tin; not more than 6% copper; and not more than 2% zinc. The second entity of amalgam is pure elemental mercury. The two components are then mixed together in a 50–50 ratio so that the end product utilized by the dentist to reconstruct your tooth is approximately 50% mercury.

There are two basic questions related to the use of amalgam. The first deals with a scientific phenomenon that results in the generation of an electrical current when two dissimilar metals are immersed or enveloped by an electrolyte fluid. In this case your saliva fulfills the role of an electrolyte and the amalgam provides dissimilar metals. Is there an electrical current being continually generated in our mouths because of this and, if so, is it causing any problems or damage? The second question is whether once the amalgam is installed in the tooth, does the material remain "locked" inside the tooth or does some of the metal escape from the tooth, in some fashion, and enter our bodies?

If some form of the involved metals does come out of the filling material and enter the body, does it cause any harm? Bearing in mind that silver, mercury, tin, and even copper can all be highly toxic to the human body systems, this book will attempt to provide you with the facts based on existing published research, so that you can make the final judgement.

Is the controversy worth reading about? Regardless of how you may ultimately judge the facts, the answer is an unqualified YES! Here is why. Those individuals that claim that the metals in the amalgam do come out and do enter the body, also claim that the following health related problems can be caused as a direct result:

BLEEDING GUMS
INCREASED SALIVATION
SOUR-METALLIC TASTE
FACIAL PARALYSIS
IRREGULAR HEARTBEAT
DEPRESSION
STRONG PAINS IN THE LEFT PART OF CHEST
RETINAL BLEEDING
DIM VISION
UNCONTROLLABLE EYE MOVEMENT
IRRITABILITY
VERTIGO
HEADACHES
JOINT PAINS
PAINS IN LOWER BACK
ETC. ETC. ETC. ETC.

Do you have any amalgam fillings in your mouth? (I estimate about 85% of the population in the United States has one or more amalgam fillings in their mouth). Have you experienced any of the above symptoms or signs? Is your interest piqued? Are you interested in your personal health and well being? Then, please read on, as the facts get much more interesting.

Sam Ziff holds a PhD in nutrition from Donsbach University in California and for the past two and a half years his work has focused exclusively on researching the potential toxicity of mercury and dental amalgam.

Mr. Ziff retired from the U.S. Air Force, with the rank of Lt. Colonel, in 1970 and has recently begun publishing a newsletter THE BIOPROBE, which provides in depth reviews of pertinent scientific literature, regarding mercury amalgam toxicity. He currently resides in Florida with is wife Helen.

CHAPTER 1

MERCURY IN MEDICINE AND DENTISTRY

Heavy metals are defined as those with the greatest atomic weights. If you haven't had chemistry that statement won't mean much to you. For our purposes, just say they are heavier than most other minerals and none have been identified as being essential to life.

The soil and water on this planet have always had some natural concentration of these metals and as a result, man has always had some exposure to them. Mineral content of soils varies greatly in different regions and, as a consquence, the first poisonings probably occurred in those areas where there was a high concentration of the heavy metals, resulting in toxic metallic contamination of the food and water supply.

Man, in his never ending struggle to improve his quality of life, has increased the metallic contamination of his environment to the point where it is the major source of heavy metal pollution and poisoning. Metals even leach out of our cookware and eating utensils. In fact, cast iron cookware used to be the major source of iron in our diets. We use constituents of these toxic heavy metals for a myriad of purposes ranging from medicines as therapeutic agents to fungicides and pesticides that we spray on the crops we grow and eat and the tobacco we may smoke.

If that wasn't sufficient, we polluted our environment with lead by the addition of tetraethyl-lead to our gasoline and burned fossil fuels like coal that contained many heavy metals including mercury. Yes, I am sure that very few of us ever realized that those huge coal-burning utility plants spew hundreds of tons of mercury out of their smoke stacks every year, year in and year out. The same is true for all the homes and factories that still burn coal.

Man in his infinite wisdom has always been capable of doing things in the name of "progress" without due regard to the impact and effect his acts or creations have on life in later years or generations of the species.

Such is truly the situation in the case of mercury utilized in medicine and dentistry. Although my concern is primarily with amalgam and dentistry, a section on the history of mercury in medicine is included just to keep everything in perspective.

I.
THE HISTORY OF MERCURY IN MEDICINE

The use of mercury in medicine predates its use in dentistry by centuries. As early as 500 B.C. there is evidence that India was using mercury as a drug. However, it appears that it was the Arabian physicians who first studied the use of mercury as a drug and introduced the use of a mercurial ointment in the 10th century.

Mercurial therapy made its way into Europe around the 13th century and spread throughout Europe. It was not widely prescribed until the 16th century. It was during this period that mercury ointments became "the drug of choice" in the treatment of syphilis. It was also in the 16th century that the controversy over the use of mercury came into focus. It was identified as the cause of poisoning among miners working in the mercury mines of Austria and Spain. The symptomatology of mercury poisoning was described as: tremor (shivering without feeling cold), gastrointestinal disturbances, oral infections, and blackening of teeth.

During the 17th century, again because of trembling, paralysis, malnutrition and premature deaths among mercury mine workers, the first standards for occupational health were introduced—the workday for mercury miners was reduced from 16 hours to 6 hours. It was also at this time that medical use of mercury seemed to fall from favor. Mercury and other metals were identified as occupational hazards for miners, gilders, chemists, potters, tinsmiths, glassworkers, mirror makers, painters, and medical personnel. There was even a law suit brought against the owner of a chemical factory that was manufacturing mercury chloride. The charge was the pollution of the local environment which contributed to an increased death rate in the neighborhood. What is really significant about this incident is that it happened in 1713 and it was one of the first public outcrys over continued use of mercury with its many adverse effects against health. Towards the end of the 17th century two important events occurred: Mercury was identified as a neurotoxicant and, in 1685, mercury nitrate began to be used in France in the preparation of fur felt, to be utilized in the making of hats.

In the 18th century, continued use of mercury therapy sparked many major controversies, especially in England. The proponents for and against took to the press to convey their positions. Regardless of the position taken, whether you were an advocate or a critic, mercury was an important topic of interest for 18th century practitioners. It was towards the end of the 18th century that the practice of prescribing mercury found its way into medical practice in the United States. Right from the outset there was controversy, intense enemies on its use as well as ardent and convinced supporters.

It was during the 19th century, that scientific experimentation with mercury began. In fact, one of the first reports on mercury's fetotoxic effects resulted from an experiment performed by Gaspard, in which he exposed fly eggs to mercury vapor in inadequate conditions of temperature and humidity. In the experimental group, no eggs hatched, whereas in the control group (not exposed to mercury vapor) hundreds of eggs hatched.

The belief that mercury cured venereal disease engendered a generalized false belief among most physicians that if mercury could cure venereal disease it could also cure other diseases that were not curable with other medicines. As a result of this false perception of mercury's efficacy its use increased dramatically during the 19th century. It became the drug of choice for almost any problem from chronic diarrhea to typhoid fever. It was also during this time that use of mercury as a diuretic agent became established as acceptable clinical practice.

Organomercurials retained their place in the modern pharmacopeia, even after several deaths as a direct result of their use and even after the introduction of other diuretics (thiazides) that did not have the toxicity of mercurials.

In the last quarter of the 19th century, French scientists discovered that mercurials possessed germicidal and antiseptic capabilities and introduced their use into clinical practice. Although side effects and deaths were reported shortly after it was introduced as an antiseptic, that didn't stop its use. In fact, a hundred years later, in 1984 you can still obtain mercurial antiseptics over the counter. The availability of pharmaceutical preparations may change in the not too distant future as the FDA is proposing the ban of all over the counter products made with mercury. This action is finally being proposed because a child recently died from using merthiolate (prescribed by her physician) to treat an infection in her ear.

During the 20th century industrial and agricultural use of mercury compounds reached their peak. There have also been some of the more severe human tragedies in the world as a result. Poisoning from mercury has caused the deaths of thousands of innocent unsuspecting people. The major incidents occurred at Minamata Bay, Japan; Northern Iraq; Guatemala; Ghana; Almagordo, New Mexico. More recently, during 1983, there were eight different incidents of Kawasaki-type disease reported from different areas of the United States to the Center for Disease Control (CDC) in Atlanta. (CDC has not concluded that mercury is the causative agent in Kawasaki disease).

The major incidents of widespread poisoning were the catalyst for focusing world-wide attention of the scientific community on the highly toxic nature of mercury and demonstrated graphically the disastrous results of human ignorance and industrial carelessness. Because of their importance to us all in understanding the insidious nature of this substance, I am going to relate in more detail some of these major incidents.

The first two incidents took place in Japan, during the period of 1953–1965. The first epidemic at Minamata Bay identified methyl mercury as the environmental contaminant involved. The second epidemic occurred in the Agano River in Niigata. In Minamata, 121 people were identified as being poisoned by methylmercury and of this number, 46 subsequently died from the poison. In Niigata there were 6 deaths out of a total of 47 cases identified as having methyl mercury poisoning. In both Minamata and Niigata the researchers were finally able to establish a relationship between the disease and the amount of fish consumed. The source of contamination to the fish was identified as the discharges from factories using mercuric chloride catalysts in the manufacture of vinyl chloride and acetaldehyde. Individuals consuming the contaminated fish suffered a generalized degenerative neurological disease. The researchers also clearly established that the mercury was penetrating the placental membrane in pregnant women and affecting the fetus. In fact the name of "Fetal Minamata Disease" was used to identify fetuses poisoned by methyl mercury because 6% of the births in Minamata resulted in children with cerebral palsy.

In Iraq there were actually three major outbreaks of alkylmercury poisoning. All involved consumption of seed grain that had been treated with either ethylmercury or methylmercury. The first outbreak occurred in 1956 and involved approximately 100 reported cases of poisoning. The second was more severe and took place in 1960. During the 1960 outbreak there were 1022 cases reported. The 1972 outbreak of methylmercury poisoning in Iraq involved over 6350 hospital admissions and certainly ranks as the worst catastrophe in the world involving toxic exposure to mercury in any form. There were 459 people who died in the hospital and whose deaths were directly attributed to their exposure to methylmercury. The predominant cause of poisoning was attributed to eating bread prepared from seed wheat that had been treated with a methylmercury fungicide. All of the classic symptoms and signs of methylmercury poisoning were present in both the adult and pediatric population who had eaten the poisoned bread.

The initial involvement of the Central Nervous System (CNS) in mercury intoxication usually produces the following symptoms: numbness and tingling of fingers, toes, nose and lips; fine tremor of the hands and usually the loss of ability to perform fine movements of the hand; there may also be a problem with walking, associated with ataxia. Ataxia is a condition involving the muscles that results in irregularity of muscular action or a failure of muscular coordination. There may also be a constriction or narrowing of the visual fields, and a loss of hearing. It was these initial symptoms that assisted in identifying mercury as the toxic agent involved. There was also an incident in the United States in 1969. In New Mexico a family of nine, including a pregnant woman, were poisoned by eating pork from animals that had been fed seed grain coated with methylmercury. This incident involved the fetus of the pregnant woman which is the only published report of fetal toxicity due to methylmercury poisoning occurring in the United States.

During 1983 there were eight different outbreaks of Kawaski disease reported in the United States. The disease is named after its discoverer Dr. Tomisaku Kawasaki, a Japanese pediatrician. During the Minamata and Niigata incidents there were about 50 cases of mucocutaneous lymph node syndrome (MLNS) that came to the attention of Dr. Kawasaki. All of these children presented with the same type of symptoms: fever of more than 5 days duration, conjunctivitis, pharyngitis (sore throat) with strawberry tongue, peripheral erythema (flushed skin) with subsequent desquamation truncal exanthem (eruptive fever and shedding of body skin) and cervical adenopathy (enlargement of lymph glands in the neck). Dr. Kawasaki published a report on his findings with the 50 cases and related it to mercury toxicity resulting from eating fish, although he was unable to confirm the presence of mercury in his patients. After publication of Dr. Kawasaki's report many other Japanese physicians realized that they had been encountering the same syndrome in many of their patients. A special MLNS study group was established under the auspices of the Japanese Ministry of Health and Welfare and between 1960 and 1976, nearly 10,000 cases were identified in Japan.

In 1974, The Pediatrics Journal published a report on MLNS by Dr. Kawasaki and his colleagues. As a result, physicians in this country became aware that the MLNS or Kawasaki disease had existed in this country since 1971. Since then more than 400 cases of MLNS occurring in the United States have been reported to the Center for Disease Control.

In one sense, we could say that there is no difference whether we talk about mercury in medicine or mercury in dentistry, both sciences use the metal therapeutically. However our problem is one of attempting to address mercury's use in dentistry rather than its role in environmental pollution or medicine. To this end, many of the facets of mercury toxicity as they relate to medicine will be addressed in the context of amalgam's relationship or possible relationship to signs and symptomatology that have been identified or established by the medical profession for specific disease states or conditions.

REFERENCES

1. Maurissen, J.P.J., History of mercury and mercurialism. New York State Journal of Medicine, Vol. 81, pages 1902–1909, 1981.

2. Almkvist, J., Some notes on the history of mercury intoxication. Acta Medica Scandinavica, Vol. 70, page 463, 1929.

3. Goldwater, L. J., From Hippocrates to Ramazzini: early history of industrial medicine. Annual Medical History, Vol. 8, page 27, 1936.

4. Francis, J. W., Observations on the natural and medical history of mercury. American Medical Recorder, Vol. 5, page 395, 1822.

5. Centers for Disease Control, Kawasaki disease. The Morbidity and Mortality Weekly Report, Vol. 29, pages 61–63, 1980, and Vol. 32, issue 7, pages 875–906, 1982–1983.

6. Bakir, F., et al. Methylmercury poisoning in Iraq. Science, Vol. 181, pages 230–241, 1973.

7. Elhassani, S. B. The many faces of methymercury poisoning. Journal of Toxicology Clinical Toxicology, Vol. 19, Issue 8, pages 98–100, 1983.

8. Goldwater, L. J. Mercury: A history of quicksilver. York Press, 1972, Baltimore, Maryland.

II.
THE HISTORY OF MERCURY IN DENTISTRY

The type of material utilized to fill teeth has always presented problems of one kind or another to the dental profession.

The ability to use any type of metal always presented difficulty to the dentist in the manipulation of it to "fill" a small area in a tooth. Over the years it was a constant challenge to the ingenuity and inventiveness of the dental practitioners to eliminate the difficulties of working with single metals to make them more pliable and capable of being molded (plastic) and which would then harden and have some permanence.

The first plastic metallic fillings, which had some quality of permanence, were called "fusible metals". D'Arcet's "mineral cement" was first in the field and was 8 parts bismuth, 5 parts lead, 3 parts tin, and $\frac{1}{10}$th part of mercury to hasten the fusing process. This was used in France and first made its appearance in the United States about 1820. The problem with this material was that it had to be melted and then poured into the cavity.

It was about 1826 that M. Taveau of Paris was advocating the use of a "Silver Paste" for permanent fillings. The silver paste proposed by M. Taveau was a simple combination of silver and mercury. For convenience sake, silver coins were subsequently used instead of the purified silver. The coins were filed down and sufficient mercury added to the filings to make a paste or plastic mass. The free mercury was then pressed out and the residue was placed in the cavity where it soon hardened.

So with the refinement of M. Taveau's silver paste by using silver coin filings which also contained other metals (like copper) used in the manufacture of the coins, silver amalgam was born and ushered into the world.

However, this new silver paste exhibited some very undesirable properties when passing from a plastic state into the rigid or hardened state. The mixture would expand after setting and it was not unusual for the patient to return with a fractured tooth or the filling protruding above the cavity, which of course would be interfering with closing of the jaw. As a result, most dentists went back to using gold foil or other substances which, although they did not have the plastic quality of amalgam, were much more preferable to the dentist than coping with the problems presented by use of the silver paste.

The ability of amalgam to be manipulated was its greatest asset and ultimately scientific experimentation would have produced an amalgam without the undesireable properties of the original formulations. I say "would have" because an incident occurred in New York City that precluded this happening for almost 60 years and, in effect, started what is commonly referred to as the 1st Amalgam War.

In 1833, two brothers by the name of Crawcour suddenly appeared in New York City and began a dental practice. They were two adventurers, who had no training, experience, or skill and who exploited the use of amalgam by an unprecedented advertising campaign. The thrust of their advertising was that they had available a new material that was much cheaper than gold and did not require the same degree of painful preparation that the use of gold did.

The professional dentists rebelled for two major reasons: 1. the exploitation and use of a filling material that was totally unsatisfactory and 2. a duty to protect the public from "charlatans". Although they were quacks, without any professional credentials, the Crawcours were fierce and ruthless competitors and soon built a thriving dental practice. In fact, they were so successful, their office was filled with the best patients of the area's foremost dentists.

This would never do, of course, so the dental profession started a relentless crusade against the foreign charlatans. Amalgam was denounced not only as a poor filling material but also as the cause of mercurial poisoning, diseases of the gums and numerous other disastrous ills. The crusade was so powerful that the Crawcours were finally compelled to retire in defeat.

The amalgam war raged within the dental profession for almost 25 additional years. Organized dentistry disowned and denounced the use of amalgam. In the forefront of the war was the American Society of Dental Surgeons founded by Dr. C. A. Harris in 1840, at about the same time he opened the first dental college in the United States, The Baltimore College of Dental Surgery.

One of the first resolutions passed by the American Society

of Dental Surgeons was to the effect that "the use of lithodeen mineral paste and all other substances of which mercury is an ingredient were hurtful both to the teeth and all parts of the mouth and that there was no tooth in which caries in it could be arrested and the organ rendered serviceable by being filled, in which gold could not be employed". Members were obliged to sign pledges promising not to use amalgam upon threat of expulsion from the Society.

Some members were actually expelled from the Society because they used amalgam. In spite of this, there was a sizeable minority, particularly those dentists working for the poorer people, who paid very little attention to the resolution. Their patients could not afford gold foil fillings, and although amalgam was an unsatisfactory filling material, it was better than anything else they could use for the fees they were able to collect.

Added to all the acrimony and bitterness was a basic resentment on the part of many of the prominent dentists of admitting that a dental society had the power to make them sign pledges or suspend them for failing to sign. In 1855, in order to put an end to the internal conflicts within the Society, most of the resolutions prohibiting use of amalgam were withdrawn. The controversy over amalgam and having its membership comply finally broke up the American Society of Dental Surgeons.

About the same time, Dr. Elisha Townsend of Philadelphia proposed an amalgam consisting of 4 parts silver and 5 parts tin which were melted together. This was then reduced to filings and mixed with mercury to make a plastic mass for use in filling cavities. Other dentists also began to experiment and develop new formulas for amalgam that hopefully would overcome the expansion problems.

Under the leadership of Dr. J. Foster Flagg, the first organized movement on behalf of amalgam was begun in the late 1870's. The movement was notable for its creed that amalgam was a valuable filling material and reports of it being injurious to the health of the patient were unfounded and untrue. Most of the experiments done to prove this new creed were inconclusive and the dental profession remained in doubt as to the advisability of using amalgam for filling teeth.

This was all changed by the efforts of one man, Dr. G. V.

Black. He spent most of his years as a teacher, lecturer, and scientific researcher. Dr. Black probably contributed more to the progress of dentistry than any other single individual. The most notable of Dr. Black's achievements was the perfection of dental amalgam in the early 1900's.

The 2nd Amalgam War started shortly thereafter and is attributed almost exclusively to the efforts of one Professor Alfred Stock of Germany. Dr. Stock taught chemistry at the Kaiser-Wilheim Institute of Chemistry, and in 1926 he elected to publish his own personal experiences with mercury, which had destroyed a major part of his life. Dr. Stock's exposure to mercury was in the laboratory in the course of teaching and chemical experimentation over 25 years.

From our standpoint, what was most significant about Dr. Stock's 1926 article, was the identification of silver amalgam fillings in the mouth as a source of mercury vapor. Moreover, he outlined the scientific experiments that confirmed his findings. Dr. Stock concluded his article with the following paragraph "Dentistry should completely avoid the use of amalgam for fillings or at least not use it whenever this is possible. There is no doubt that many symptoms: tiredness, depression, irritability, vertigo, weak memory, mouth inflamations, diarrhea, loss of appetite and chronic catarrhs often are caused by mercury which the body is exposed to from amalgam fillings, in small amounts, but continuously. Doctors should give this fact their serious consideration. It will then likely be found that the thoughtless introduction of amalgam as a filling material for teeth was a severe sin against humanity".

With that article started the second amalgam war. Charges and counter charges were the order of the day and this continued on (in fact it's still going on) until events of World War II temporarily halted the arguments. Stock continued his research, and in 1939 published an article outlining further facts about amalgam. He identified it as an unstable alloy that continuously gave off mercury in the form of gas ions and abraded particles. Stock's articles created consternation among the metallurgists, doctors, dentists, and chemists and were reported in great detail in the press. Dr. Frykholm states that at a lecture in Sweden in 1941, Stock modified his position by claiming that the rare cases of mercury poisoning caused by mercury vapor leaching out of amalgam restorations should not affect the further use of silver amalgam in dental practice. This appears to be an error or misinterpretation made by Dr. Frykholm in the translation of that speech. In another translation made by Mats Hanson and stated in a presentation he made at a seminar on mercury toxicity given in Colorado in September of 1983, Hanson stated that Stock reaffirmed his position that amalgam was highly toxic and should not be used by the dental profession as a restoration material.

Whose translation is correct is immaterial because all of Stock's research findings related to amalgam and mercury have essentially been confirmed. The latest in 1984.

After World War II, the world went about the business of picking up the pieces and getting on with life. However, it wasn't long before the continued use of mercury in dentistry evoked those same passionate pro or con amalgam positions within the dental and scientific communities. Behind it all of course was Stock's work and the burning questions raised by him: Does mercury actually escape from dental amalgam fillings? If it does escape, does it do any damage to the human body?

Enter the "3rd Amalgam War". A war that is still in progress and will continue on until organized dentistry, medicine, and "the establishment" either accept the anti-amalgam position with its overwhelming array of documented scientific research or, once and for all times, provide incontrovertible proof that mercury in amalgam does not escape from the filling material once it is in the tooth or, that if any mercury does escape that it is not toxic to the human body in continuous micro dosages.

The battle was joined, on many fronts and in many countries of the world. In order for you to have a better grasp of some of the battles and on what battlefields they were and are being fought the following overview is provided.

The American Dental Association which came into being at about the same time the American Society of Dental Surgeons was being dissolved, supported the use of silver amalgam then as the restoration material of choice and still does today. I suppose Psychiatrists or Psychologists might be able to explain why certain officials of this fine professional association adhere so vehemently to a policy that continues to champion the use of mercury amalgam. Or they might advance some acceptable rationale that would also explain why these same individuals go out of their way to denigrate the use of non-toxic replacement materials for posterior restorations, when such materials are available today and in fact, are comparable or superior to amalgam.

I wholeheartedly champion the doctrine of reasonable doubt. The scientific community should take a lesson from the courts of law in this regard and if there is a reasonable doubt that a substance may be injurious to the human organism, its use should be stopped. It just doesn't make sense to continue the use of a product that is known to be one of the most toxic to man when there are suitable substitutes that at this point in time can be considered non-toxic.

In regard to the use of composite materials for posterior restorations there seems to be a double standard being applied by the ADA in accepting materials for inclusion in their list of approved filling materials. The new composites are being subjected to very rigid standards requiring up to seven years of testing in the mouth in addition to meeting the basic structural requirements. Conversely, it appears that new amalgam formulations are being approved if they meet the structural requirements, as over 100 different amalgams are on their approved list. If each required 7 years of testing I don't think any of them could survive the wait.

This lack of acceptance of the newer composites by the ADA has some serious overtones. Insurance companies are using this fact to deny payment of claims where the dentist has used the new composites for posterior restorations. This is truly an unfortunate situation which only hurts the patient. The new composites show greater structural strength than amalgam and have exhibited wear characteristics that are close to that of amalgam.

I was always under the impression that it was the dentist who went to college to learn his profession and that once he had graduated and had been licensed to practice dentistry in his particular state, it was the dentist's decision how best to treat his patient. I must be wrong because we now have the situation where the insurance companies and the ADA determine what the dentist can do. It is not price that the insurance companies are objecting to but rather that the composite materials being used for posterior restorations are not on the ADA list of approved materials.

The ADA also appears to have some problem in accepting the findings of some research papers. Articles published in non-United States scientific journals do not seem to command the same attention and acceptance than those articles published in U.S. Journals do. That is with the exception of those articles that support the ADA position on mercury amalgam.

It is extremely interesting that any scientific article refuting Stock's work seems to be acceptable to the ADA while the great volume of scientific evidence confirming Stock's work is ignored or the implications are that the research was flawed.

This is especially true when you consider that the major work of Dr. Karl O. Frykholm, published in Acta Odontologica Scandinavica in Stockholm Sweden in 1957, has been the cornerstone of the American Dental Association's policy that amalgam is safe except in those few individuals who may be hypersensitive to mercury. All of the published articles based on experiments that utilized much more sophisticated equipment than that used by Dr. Frykholm and which arrived at conclusions contrary to Frykholm's have been totally ignored by the ADA, or interpreted in such a manner that the conclusions supported the ADA position.

REFERENCES

1. History of dental and oral science in America, prepared under direction of the American Academy of Dental Science, Published by Samuel S. White, 1876, Philadelphia, Pennsylvania.

2. Bremmer, D. K., The Story of Dentistry, revised 3rd edition, 1954. Dental Items of Interest Publishing Co., Inc., Brooklyn, N.Y.

3. Stock, A., The Hazards of Mercury Vapor. Zeitsch Angew Chem, Vol. 39, pages 461–488, 1926.

4. Hanson, M., Nothing New Under The Sun: Experiences with Mercury Poisoning Related by Dr. Alfred Stock and Dr. E. Jaensch in 1926. Journal of Orthomolecular Psychiatry, Vol. 12, issue 3, pages 355–358, 1983.

5. Frykholm, K. O., On Mercury from Dental Amalgam: Its Toxic and Allergic Effects and some Comments on Occupational Hygiene. Acta Odontologica Scandanivica, Vol. 22, Supplement 22, pages 1–123, 1957.

6. Flagg, J. F., The Choice of Proper Filling Material, 1900.

CHAPTER 2

WHERE ARE WE NOW?

You should be made aware of the magnitude of the problems related to research and the dissemination of research findings. The type of research we are speaking of involves those areas that have the potential to impact on man as a species and to affect his survival.

The complexity of the problem is mind boggling. To place it in some sort of perspective, let's look at the problem of heart disease and take the thousands of papers that have been published on this particular subject as an example:

Problem 1. These papers have been published in hundreds of different journals and books all over the world.

Problem 2. There is no universal language for the publication of scientific research. Consequently, if a Russian scientist should publish his findings on an aspect of heart disease that has taken years of scientific experimentation, it would be written in Russian and published in a Russian journal or book. It might languish there for years until some other government, company, or individual discovers it and ascertains it is worthy of translation into their language. Here in the United States, a great percentage of this translation is done under sponsorship of the concerned agency of the federal government. It is then published by the U.S. Government Printing Office and made available to the public at a price. How does Dr. Jones the cardiologist practicing in Los Angeles, know that the government has just published a major Russian research work on heart disease? The only way he would ever find out is if one of the American journals he subscribes to happened to have a researcher and/or reporter who became aware of the translated Russian paper and thought it was significant enough to do an article about it.

Problem 3. The average health professional usually subscribes to all of the publications related to his specialty or particular area of interest. Finding time to read them is another matter. Some have their staff skim the articles and point out the ones that they should read. Others just pile them up in stacks, promising themselves they will take time to go through them. His time is taken up not only in attending to his patients, but he is actually running a business and must devote a percentage of his time to business matters. Then there is his family and social obligations and the requirement to attend seminars or formal classes that are a part of his profession's continuing education requirement to maintain professional standing. Last, but not least, there is always the spector of a malpractice suit hanging over his head and additional time must be spent in insuring everything that could have been done, has in fact been done.

Problem 4. If an individual had nothing to do except read 12 hours a day, it would probably take him six months to find and read everything that was published TODAY that pertained to his specialty or area of interest. By the time he finished reading the information published today, it would have been updated or superseded by hundreds of other articles.

Problem 5. The answer to a problem may be obscured. There are literally thousands of enzyme systems in the body. A team of 5 medical doctors and biochemists have just spent 2 years researching one enzyme system. They have documented everything it does and how it does it and its interrelationships to various other functions and organs, glands, blood, muscles, etc. etc.. They have also determined which amino acids, vitamins, minerals, hormones, etc., are affected by this enzyme. Truly a remarkable and historical research effort. However, unknown to them, another team of researchers is investigating the impact of various drugs (normally prescribed) on this same particular enzyme system. Their results indicate that if you take Drug A, it will inhibit the enzyme from performing its normal functions. What they didn't know was that still another group, testing the same drug, reached a conclusion that it had no effect at all on that particular enzyme system. Confused? Wait! The three reports are published individually in three different journals, only one of which your doctor subscribes to. Wait!!! There is more. As soon as the article is published, doctors and scientists all over the world who are familiar with the subject and/or have been doing their own independent research, write in and either point out what they consider to be flaws in the basic protocol used for the research, or tell of their own experiences using the drug, which are contrary to the information published. If your doctor had only read one of the articles, how could he make an informed judgment? That analogy would apply to a great many of today's dentists who continue to use mercury amalgam fillings. They have just not been exposed to the preponderance of scientific data that would permit them to make a rational personal judgement on the subject.

Problem 6. Don't bother me with the facts! The high ego, authoritarian health professional will sometimes find published articles so contrary to his training and beliefs that he totally closes his mind to the fact that they might be true. Can you blame him? What would you do if you had spent from 5 to 14 years studying a particular way of doing something and you were even recognized as an expert in your field, and suddenly you are confronted with evidence done in a laboratory with test tubes and animals that implies everything you have been doing and advocating is wrong? I am sure you would resist or even try to set up research projects to prove you weren't wrong, or to find evidence refuting the findings contrary to your own. How can you blame the physician, who received 3 hours of instruction on nutrition out of 8 years of formal training, for laughing when you ask him whether nutrition would help cure your particular problem. By the same token, how can you blame your dentist for putting silver amalgam in your mouth when it has been used for over 150 years for that very purpose? In both instances it is only in recent years that researchers have had available to them large computerized data bases that have permitted the review and correlation of data from multiple disciplines. Even with the data available, it is an awesome task correlating information from biochemistry, chemistry, metallurgy, electrochemistry, pathology, physiology, neurology, pharmacology, toxicology, etc., and then interpreting and assembling the results of your research into cohesive statements. For example, the information upon which this book is being written, is based on research articles compiled over a 2½ year span.

Problem 7. How do you ascertain if something proven in a laboratory with sophisticated analytical machinery, test tubes, chemicals, and animals is true in the human body? Fortunately, you can't go around killing human beings and dissecting and assaying their bodies. Therefore, some things can never be proven to the satisfaction of the pure scientist. As a rule, the scientific world does not accept anecdotal evidence as proof. What this means is that if you had a serious health problem and took a particular vitamin, or performed a certain type of exercise, or only ate certain foods and you got better, that would be an anecdote and not a scientific fact. To be scientific you would have to have a double blind study. This is where two groups of patients are established, all with similar symptoms and all within the same age grouping. One group is given placebos (sugar pills) and the other is given the actual vitamin. Neither group nor the investigators knows what they are taking. At the end of the test period, the results are analyzed and a conclusion is drawn from the results as to the efficacy of the vitamin.

Why have I belabored the problems related to research? The answer is quite simple—our current situation with silver amalgam. There is a substantial flow of anecdotal evidence being reported by dentists and physicians who believe that the research to date has indicated with sufficient clarity that amalgams in teeth may be injurious to our health. These health practitioners have recommended removal of amalgam fillings and replacement with new composite materials (composed of quartz or other fillers and certain plastic compounds) that are basically non-toxic. Where the patient has agreed to this type of reconstruction and the work was performed, there has usually been an abatement, amelioration or complete clearing of symptoms. This is not true in all cases because here again we are dealing with the most complex piece of machinery in the world, "The Human Body", and we are all different biochemically. Questions such as: How long has the problem existed? Has irreparable damage been done which cannot be corrected by removing or correcting the cause of the problem? Is there another cause existant at the same time? And on and on.

On the other side of the problem we have the proponents who advocate continued use of amalgam fillings. The combined credentials and strength of this group is awesome. It includes the National Institute of Dental Research, National Bureau of Standards, The American Dental Association (ADA), The Academy of General Dentistry (AGD), most of the state dental societies, all of the teaching college and university dental schools and most of the medical doctors. Although the ADA in reality is only a professional association, they in effect set the acceptable standards for the dental industry.

Of the 100,000 plus practicing dentists in the United States, there is only a small minority at this time (somewhere in the order of 2000) who do not accept the ADA position on the use of amalgam in dentistry. The official ADA position on this problem as expressed in the Journal of the American Dental Association, Vol 106, April, 1983, is summarized in the following quote: "The Association wishes to emphasize that except in individuals sensitive to mercury, there is no reason why a patient should seek at this time to have amalgam restorations (silver fillings) removed. Indeed, the effect of such a procedure and further restorative operations could be detrimental to the patients oral health, including the unnecessary loss of teeth and cannot be justified." There are several things about that statement that bother me, not the least of which is the question of for whom the article was being written? Doesn't it seem kind of strange that in a professional journal for dentists, the "unnamed authors" would have to parenthetically explain to the doctors that amalgam restorations meant "silver fillings"???

The last point aside, you can see that we do have a real conflict and difference of opinion. Each side is armed with published scientific research, in many instances the same research, that is being interpreted as supporting their position.

WHAT TO DO?

The balance of this book will try to tell the story of the research that has been published. We will try to relate, in terms and language that a non-technical person can understand, both sides of the debate and let you be the final judge. Your decision may be influenced to some degree by your own health status and whether anyone up till now has been able to give you a satisfactory answer as to what is causing your condition or problem, if you have a health condition or problem.

CHAPTER 3

WHAT IS MERCURY?

At this point, it is extremely important to attempt to define what mercury or quicksilver (as it is sometimes called) really is.

Mercury is a highly toxic silver-white, liquid metal which is highly volatile at ordinary temperatures and the fumes of which are readily absorbed when inhaled.

Is all mercury toxic or injurious to our health? The answer is an unqualified yes. Some forms of this metal are much more toxic than others. In this book we will deal with the two main groupings of mercury compounds, inorganic and organic.

INORGANIC MERCURY

Within this group there is: elemental mercury, elemental mercury vapor, elemental mercurous and mercuric salts and some complexes of the mercuric ions that can form reversible bonds with certain tissue ligands such as thiol groups on protein. The last statement merely means that once inside your body, the mercury can attach itself to sulfur containing compounds that are part of a protein molecule. In other words it is a hitchhiker who has caught a ride on a vehicle that is part of a pretty sophisticated transport system that travels to all parts of our bodies.

We can absorb inorganic mercury by inhalation of the vapor from elemental mercury or aerosols of mercuric salts. It can enter orally or be absorbed through the skin, mucous membranes and digestive tract.

Elemental mercury is the most volatile form of the metal because it readily gives off vapor when agitated, compressed, heated, or exposed to the air at normal temperature. Elemental mercury is used in dentistry to make the silver amalgam fillings. It is also found in barometers, thermometers and medical instruments. Our concern with elemental mercury relates to any exposure to the vapors given off, because the vapor is so readily absorbed by our bodies when inhaled. Diffusion of elemental mercury vapor into the tissues and across cell membranes is facilitated by its lipid solubility (will mix with fats) and its lack of an electrical charge. The electrical charge, whether positive or negative, has a lot to do with how different materials get in and out of our cells to do the jobs nature designed for them.

Mercurous Chloride is the best known of the mercurous compounds. It is sometimes referred to as Calomel which for years was used as a cathartic but is not used anymore. It is, however, still used in some skin creams as an antiseptic. Mercurous Iodide was once used as a treatment for syphilis.

Mercuric salts are a very irritating and toxic form of the metal. Mercuric chloride is used as an antiseptic and is very toxic when swallowed. In fact, it is so toxic that it was one of the preferred poisons with which to commit suicide with. Mercurochrome and thiomersal (merthiolate) utilized as antiseptics are considered by the medical profession to be relatively safe because of the dilute solution and the fact that the solution is less soluble and doesn't penetrate the skin easily. Once again, current information is drastically changing this opinion. The FDA has recently published an advisory concerning the death of a child who was being treated with merthiolate for an infection in her ear. As a result, the FDA is now proposing regulatory change that would forbid the use of mercury in any over-the-counter product.

Mercuric salts are still widely employed in industry today. Waste from these industries is discharged into nearby rivers, thus polluting them in many parts of the world.

Continued exposure to mercuric salts can cause neurological and behavioral changes. The phrase "He is Mad as a

Hatter" and the character of the Mad Hatter in Lewis Carrol's Alice's Adventures in Wonderland, stem from the "changes" that used to happen to people who worked in the felt hat industry. If you recall, in the chapter on medical history, we said that an important event occurred towards the end of the 17th century. In 1685, mercury nitrate began to be used in France in the preparation of fur felt. The mercury nitrate was used in the carrotting process in making fur felt for the hats.

ORGANIC MERCURY

This group of compounds are also called organomercurials and as with the inorganic mercury, toxicity varies depending upon the particular compound. Within this grouping alkylmercurials are considered the most dangerous. They can enter the body by inhalation, skin absorption or oral ingestion. They are volatile and exposure to their vapors can readily occur. They are also lipid soluble (this means they will dissolve in fats normally available in our bodies) and readily cross biological membranes making for highly toxic potentials.

Alkylmercury salts have been widely used as fungicides. Use as such has led to major incidents of human poisoning from the inadvertent consumption of mercury treated seed grain. The worst incident occurred in Iraq in 1972. Wheat and barley seed grain that had been treated with methylmercury was distributed for use in planting only. Instead, the grain was ground into flour and made into bread. As a result, approximately 6500 people were hospitalized and 500 died.

Methylmercury is very volatile. So much so that it is chemically reduced to be used as a liquid or solid aerosol spray. When inhaled in the form of aerosols, these compounds are likely to dissolve quickly in body fluids and be distributed to the blood.

Phenyl mercuric propionate is used as an antimildew additive. It is incorporated in many of the water based paints used on exteriors. It is a potentially dangerous source of mercury intoxication that could result from inhalation of its toxic vapors.

To give you some idea of the overall mercury pollution problem, let's look at the following facts:

CHLORINE AND ALKALI PRODUCERS. For every ton of chlorine produced, nearly half a pound of mercury escapes into the environment. This adds up to about 1,200,000 pounds a year.

AGRICULTURE. About 1,000,000 pounds a year are used as fungicides protecting our seed grains and as insecticides spraying our plants.

COAL BURNING. The average mercury content of coal is about 0.3 parts per million. Of this, approximately 95% is expelled in flue gases during combustion. World atmospheric contamination by coal burning is estimated to be about 6–10 million lbs. per year.

VOLCANOES. Mercury also enters the world oceans from this source.

Overall, it is estimated that 20,000,000 pounds of mercury flow into the sea each year, half of this of natural origin and the other half from industrial sources. It would take years to document all of the industrial users of mercury around the world and calculate their contributions to the overall pollution problem. I think it would be safe to assume that the foregoing information represents only the tip of the iceberg.

So far, we have provided little information relating to the main purpose of writing this book. It is not a crusade against mercury per se but is intended to forcefully bring out the point that our total body burden of mercury can come from many sources. The fact has a very specific relationship to be considered by you when making your final judgement about the dental and medical professions use of mercury.

Do dentists use a a lot of mercury? Present estimates are that approximately 250,000 lbs. a year are being used in the U.S. alone and that by the year 2000, this figure could be 600,000 lbs. That's a lot of mercury going into the mouths/bodies of human beings.

As we have stated previously, our major health concern really centers around inhaling vapours from elemental mercury and methylmercury vapor from organic mercury. The heart of the controversy swirling around the use of silver amalgam as a dental filling material, is the essential and critical answer which you as an individual with mercury amalgam fillings in your mouth must reach is: "Has my personal health or the health of my family been adversely affected because of these controversial fillings?'' So that YOU and not some un-named committee of an association can make this important decision, the following chapter will attempt to provide you with all the arguments being used FOR and AGAINST the continued use of mercury amalgam as the desired dental filling material.

REFERENCES

1. Arena, J. M., Poisoning, 4th edition, 1979, Charles C. Thomas, Springfield, Illinois, 1979.

2. Goodman and Gillman's, The Pharmacological Basis of Therapeutics, 6th edition, 1980, The Macmillan Publishing Co., Inc., New York.

3. Safety of Dental Amalgam, Journal American Dental Association, 106:74–76, 1983.

4. Seese, W. S., and Daub, G. H., Basic Chemistry, 2nd Edition, 1977, Prentice-Hall, Inc., Englewood Cliffs, N.J.

5. Dickey, L. D. (Ed), Clinical Ecology, Charles C. Thomas, Springfield, Illinois, 1976.

6. Billings, C. E., and Matson, W. R., Mercury Emissions from Coal Combustion, Science, 176:1232, 1972.

7. Schroeder, H. S., The Poisons Around Us, Keats Publishing, New Canaan, CT., 1974.

8. Land Yearbook, U.S. Department of Agriculture, 1958.

9. Minerals Yearbook, U.S. Bureau of Mines, 1972.

10. A Recommended Standard for Occupational Exposure to Inorganic Mercury, USDHEW, Public Health Service, National Institute for Occupational Safety and Health (NIOSH), 1973.

CHAPTER 4

THE ARGUMENTS FOR AND AGAINST

The FOR position as expressed in each one of the following arguments represents a position of the American Dental Association and/or the proponents of continued use of amalgam that are referenced by the ADA, and/or those research papers that the ADA has interpreted to be supportive of their position. Where available I have cited the scientific references used as a basis for the ADA position taken.

I should point out at this time an idiosyncrasy of the ADA that disturbs me. The No-Author/No-Name position/policy papers published by the ADA. Most of the important decisions and policies published by the ADA in their Journal or Newspaper show the author as the "Council on Dental Materials, Instruments and Equipment; Council on Dental Therapeutics; or Bureau of Economic Research and Statistics". I should think that of the more than 100,000 dentists who are members of the ADA, someone would complain and insist that the names of the Council or Bureau members (certainly the Chairman or Head) be printed in the article or in each issue. Certainly the dentists, or at the very least we the patients, are entitled to know who (and even possibly what their qualifications are) is making all of these decisions for an entire profession that can have such a bearing on the health of an entire population.

It is paradoxical that the dentists of 1850 rebelled against their Association, The American Society of Dental Surgeons, because the Society was attempting to dictate to them what filling material they could use. Here we are in 1984, and nobody seems to be questioning the right of the American Dental Association to dictate to them; not even those whose voices are raised in protest against the continued use of amalgam. Their fight is against the use of amalgam and not the right of a professional association to dictate policy.

Immediately following the FOR positions, I have listed the AGAINST positions. These are the answers derived only from published scientific research papers, articles, or books, that can be considered as reflecting conclusions contrary to those taken by the American Dental Association. The information contained in the AGAINST positions essentially represents the facts being used by those dentists who have made their individual decisions to stop using mercury amalgam in their dental practice.

You, the reader, must be the final judge of which position is right or wrong because, in the end, it is you who should make the important decision: "YES", please put some more poison in my body because I agree with you that there really isn't a reasonable doubt that it can harm me in any way. Or "NO", there is enough evidence it can harm me. The burden of proof is on you and not me. You must prove to my satisfaction that it is safe to put in my body. The doctrine of reasonable doubt must prevail. If you cannot prove beyond a reasonable doubt that the mercury you want to put in my mouth will not be damaging to my body now or at some future date, then I must insist that you do not place more amalgam fillings in my mouth. I would also like you to remove and replace my existing mercury amalgam fillings with something other than a known poison. I understand that you cannot provide me with unequivocal scientific proof that mercury is not harming my body. However, because it is my body, I am willing to accept "anecdotal" evidence as proof of reasonable doubt!

ARGUMENT 1
THE AMERICAN DENTAL ASSOCIATION IS CONSTANTLY STUDYING AND EVALUATING THE SAFETY AND TOLERANCE OF MERCURY USED IN DENTAL RESTORATIONS

SOURCE: Journal of the American Dental Association (JADA), Vol 106, April 1983.

TITLE: Safety of Dental Amalgam

AUTHOR: Council on Dental Materials, Instruments and Equipment

Council on Dental Therapeutics

STATEMENT: "The Councils have received several inquiries regarding the continued use of dental amalgam and the practice by some of removing amalgam restorations and replacing them with gold alloy castings or composite restorative materials. Dental amalgam is used in approximately 75% of the single tooth restorations. The use of mercury in these restorations is constantly being studied and evaluated for its safety and tolerance."

FOR: The last sentence in the statement puts forth a policy position that the ADA is constantly studying the use of mercury in restorations for safety and tolerance. Unfortunately, the ADA cites no references to indicate research that the association has done and/or sponsored to support the policy position. As a result I can only conclude that the Council assumes their normal conduct of business reflects that position.

AGAINST: I was unable to find any published research finding of primary research that had been done by the ADA. However further along in the source article, the ADA states that they have two existing programs to investigate the effects of high levels of mercury vapor on the health of dental personnel. These programs are not designed to investigate the potential toxic effects of dental amalgam fillings. They are only designed to measure the amount of mercury in the urine of participating dentists associated with their exposure to mercury in their normal work environment. As for safety and tolerance in the patient, they cite (elsewhere in the source article) an article published in the June 1982 issue of the California Dental Association Journal, which consisted of a review of existing literature. This particular article presents evidence which appears to be contrary to the authors' conclusions which stated that the use of amalgams in fillings is relatively safe.

I am unable to judge what is the exact meaning of the term "relatively safe," in its application to the health of hundreds of millions of people.

ARGUMENT 2
DENTISTRY NEED ONLY CONCERN ITSELF WITH THE POTENTIAL TOXICITY OF MERCURY VAPOR

SOURCE: JADA, Vol 106, April 1983.
TITLE: Safety of Dental Amalgam.
AUTHOR: Council on Dental Materials, Instruments and Equipment
Council on Dental Therapeutics
STATEMENT: "An international committee on the hazards of mercury, classified mercury and it compounds in the order of their decreasing toxicity: first, methyl and ethyl mercury compounds, next mercury vapor, and last the inorganic salts as well as a number of organic forms. The toxic potential of these forms of mercury in dentistry is limited to mercury vapor."
FOR: Here again, the ADA does not cite any references to support the last sentence which is their policy position. I would have to assume that they are basing their statement on the work of Dr. K. O. Frykholm published in 1957. Dr. Frykholm concluded from his experiments that a small transient amount of mercury vapor escapes from newly installed amalgam fillings but that it only lasts for about a week and is not a problem. Which would then leave the main focus of the ADA's concern to be the mercury vapor that may be present in the dental office environment. There concern here centers around the fact that the elemental mercury utilized to make the amalgam is highly volatile and gives off mercury vapor when exposed to normal room temperature which is increased during the normal process of handling and mixing. In this regard, the ADA has been extremely effective in educating dental personnel as to the hazards of mercury vapor and has published many fine articles on the subject over the years.

AGAINST: The classification of the different forms of mercury in their order of toxicity is correct. The statement concerning dentistry's concern being only with mercury vapor is incorrect. Dentistry must be concerned with methylmercury, the most toxic of the various forms of mercury, because of biological processes that can transform the mercury vapor in the body into methyl mercury. These processes are biotransformation and methylation.

Biotransformation: Elemental mercury (this is the kind used in dentistry) produces mercury vapor. This fact has never been disputed. What has always been questioned is that mercury amalgam once installed in a tooth gives off mercury vapor. Dr. Stock demonstrated this in 1926 and published papers detailing his experiments and findings. Dr. Stock's original findings have been confirmed by several researchers the latest of which are: Dr. Gay and associates in 1979; Dr. Reinhardt and associates in 1979; and Dr. Svare and associates in 1981. These groups of researchers measured the amount of mercury vapor in the mouth before and after chewing gum for 10 minutes and have produced scientific proof that amalgams give off mercury vapor during the normal processes of chewing and swallowing.

Now we have established the fact that there is a continuous source of mercury vapor. When mercury vapor is inhaled there is a very rapid and efficient absorption of it by the lungs. Depending upon the amount being inhaled, the absorption rate can be from 74% for large amounts and up to 100% for small amounts. (Berlin, et al, 1969, Kudak, F. Nielsen 1965). Once absorbed, about 30% of the mercury vapor is transferred to the blood within 10 minutes. (Berlin, et al, 1969).

It is at this point that biotransformation begins. Some of the mercury vapor remains unchanged and some of it is oxidized. (This means to remove a pair of hydrogen atoms and to combine with oxygen. Chemically it means the increase of a positive electrical charge and the decrease of the negative charge which in effect ionizes the vapor). The unchanged portion exists dissolved in the blood lipids (fats). The toxic effects are produced by that portion that is oxidized into mercuric ions which occurs partly in the blood, partly in the tissues but mainly in the erythrocytes (which most of us know by the more common name of red blood cells or corpuscles). (Clarkson, 1972).

Where does methylation come in? This presents a much more technical set of circumstances and involves organisms and bacteria found in the mouth and in the gut. It all begins with the amalgam filling in the mouth. Once installed in your tooth, there are several different factors that impact on the longevity of the filling: chewing, which exerts a tremendous compaction pressure and also tends to generate heat; saliva, which represents the acid level of your oral fluids which are also considered as electrolytes—the dissimilar metals contained in the amalgam are capable of generating electrical current between themselves and/or between adjacent filled teeth or teeth with crowns made of gold or other metal; then there are the problems associated with the acids contained in many of the foods we like to eat and drink, especially coffee, tea, and colas and the increased heat from hot liquids, foods and smoking, causing an increase in the vaporization. The filling, made of an unstable alloy to start with, is subjected to all of these various factors and forces. It begins to corrode and, as a result, not only continually gives off mercury in the form of vapor but also as mercuric ions and abraded particles. So we now have transport of a portion of the mercury into the stomach along with the food and liquid.

Several researchers, beginning with Jernelov in 1969, have demonstrated the microbial conversion or methylation of mercury by various microorganisims. This was demonstrated in the laboratory as well as inside the bodies of animals (Abdulla, et al 1973). In 1975, the methylation of mercuric chloride in human feces was demonstrated by Edwards and McBride. It was also in 1975 that Rowland, Grasso and Davies determined that most strains of staphlylococci, streptococci, yeasts and escherichiacoli found in the human intestine (these are bacteria and yeasts of different forms and shapes that are normally present in the human gut) were capable of methylating mercury. It was in 1983 that Heintze and his associates made the startling discovery that various forms of oral streptococci common in dental plaque and saliva could also methylate mercury being released from the amalgam fillings.

Based on the above stated facts, I must conclude that the ADA policy position regarding dentistry being concerned only with mercury vapor is incorrect.

ARGUMENT 3
RECENT TEST INDICATING THE RELEASE OF MERCURY VAPOR FROM DENTAL AMALGAMS IN TEETH MAY NOT BE VALID

SOURCE: JADA, Vol 106, April 1983.
TITLE: Safety of Dental Amalgam
AUTHOR: Council on Dental Materials, Instruments and Equipment
Council on Dental Therapeutics.

STATEMENT: "The dental profession is continuously evaluating the implications of exposure to mercury vapor. This attention is stimulated by the potential "body burden" of mercury from food and other sources along with the accumulations from dental treatment. The release of mercury vapor from dental amalgam in the mouth has recently been reported. (1) This information was obtained with measuring devices that show detectable amounts of mercury vapor in expired air which was collected immediately after chewing on old as well as new amalgam restorations. The authors do not indicate that the air was exhaled through the nose or mouth. If through the mouth, there is no evidence that the measurable mercury vapor was from the lungs or just the oral cavity." (The footnoted reference [1] is the article by Dr. Svare and associates published in Sept. 1981).

FOR: The "body burden" of mercury derived from our food supply and other sources is certainly a major cause for continued concern. Although no references were cited by the ADA, there have been a great number of studies done that indicate in the normal course of eating and breathing we can contribute to our total body burden of mercury. The significance of whether measurements were made while the test patients were breathing through their nose or mouth relates to the basic fact that by breathing through the nose, no air from the lungs would be passing through the oral cavity and the measurement of any mercury vapor present would accurately reflect any vapor coming from amalgams. Conversley, if the patients were breathing through their mouth, the measurements might be contaminated by vapor being expired from the lungs.

AGAINST: The Councils appear to be making some valid points in their statement. However, and for your benefit, let's take a close look at the statement sentence by sentence and really see what they are saying. "The dental profession is continuously evaluating the implications of exposure to mercury vapor. This attention is stimulated by the potential "body burden" of mercury from food and other sources along with any accumulations from dental treatment." When the Councils use the phrase the "dental profession", I personally have a serious problem in attempting to determine who in the dental profession is being stimulated by the potential body burden from food and other sources. Although not referenced directly in the source document, the ADA appears to be indirectly (through the article published by Drs. Bauer and First) referencing the work of Dr. Stofen, published in the Toxicology Journal in 1974, to support their position. In this article, Dr. Stofen states that even though mercury may be released from amalgam restorations, the amount is equal to the amount ingested through food consumption and is therefore of little concern. The rationale behind this comparison eludes me. It could mean that if one ounce of poison doesn't appear to do any damage then certainly two ounces won't harm you either.

The last part of the second sentence also addresses accumulations from dental treatment. I don't know what the Councils mean by that statement except by implication. I do know that over the years their official position has been that the patient is only exposed while the restoration is being placed in the mouth. This position, I am assuming, is based on the findings of Dr. Frykholm who concluded that mercury vapor was only released from new fillings for 5 days. After that time the filling had hardened and sealed and did not constitute a problem. By "accumulation" they must mean only those mercury particles and mercury vapor present during the first five days. That seems to be a correct interpretation because in their next three sentences they imply that the research indicating mercury is released from old fillings is flawed and that the mercury vapor measured was probably being exhaled from the lungs of the patients being tested. What this leaves the reader with is an impression that we normally exhale mercury everytime we breathe; which in some of us may be true. (A complete analysis of Dr. Frykholm's article will be provided in subsequent arguments).

This leaves us with only the problem of examining the validity of Dr. Svare's findings, and the questioning of them by the ADA. Dr. Svare's article was published in the Journal of Dental Research, Vol 60, Sept. 1981. His co-authors Drs. Reinhardt, Petersen, Boyer, Frank, Gay and Cox, had all been involved since 1978 in testing the hypothesis that amalgam restorations release mercury vapor. To a large degree, these researchers were validating the findings of Dr. Stock published in 1926. They were confirming his findings through exact measurements utilizing advanced instrumentation designed solely for the purpose of measuring the mercury vapor content of air. More importantly, they were able to gain these measurements in experiments that parallel normal use of our teeth; i.e., chewing and not chewing.

The design of the experiment involved the taking of mercury vapor measurements, or readings, in the mouth before chewing and after chewing gum for 10 minutes. There were two groups of test patients in the experiment: the controls, or individuals without any fillings of any kind in their mouths, and the second group of patients who all had amalgam fillings in their teeth. In the control group without fillings, the researchers were able to detect very small amounts of mercury vapor before chewing gum. After chewing gum for 10 minutes, the amount of mercury vapor measured in the expired breath remained the same—NO CHANGE. In the test group with amalgam fillings in their teeth, measureable amounts of mercury vapor were detected before they began chewing gum. After chewing gum for 10 minutes the researchers discovered a 15.5-fold increase in the amount of mercury vapor in their breath.

It seems that Dr. Svare and his associates demonstrated in a very clear concise way that mercury vapor is continuously being released in the mouth and that this condition is greatly aggravated by the normal processes of chewing or eating. The ADA or the Councils would have us believe by the way the policy position is phrased, that the mercury was really being exhaled out of the lungs and not being released from the amalgam filled teeth. If that were true, then the researchers should have been able to duplicate the results in the mouths of those people who had no fillings because that is what the ADA is in effect saying. Which, of course the study showed could not be done.

Even without the fact that there were no changes in the readings within the control group, the ADA offers no logical explanation as to why the group with amalgams had an increased amount of mercury vapor in their breath. Certainly they don't want us to believe that the simple act of chewing gum increases the release of mercury from our lungs. Or do they?

It is quite possible that the Councils' basic assumption put forth in the statement was founded in the fact that scientific experiments have demonstrated that a percentage of an ingested dose of mercury is exhaled in the lungs. One such experiment was conducted by Drs. Hursh, Clarkson, Cherian, Vostal and Vandermallie in 1976. In their study, they exposed 5 human volunteers to radioactive mercury vapor and concluded: the subjects retained an average of 74% of the mercury inhaled; of the 74% that was retained in the body, 7% was lost in the expired air and that the half-life of the retained mercury was 18 hours.

The term half-life is utilized to define the length of time required for living tissue or organisms to eliminate one-half of a radioactive substance which has been introduced into the body. The remaining half will have the same half-life as the original. This means that in their experiment, every 18 hours one-half of the amount remaining will be eliminated. For example, if the 74% retained amounted to 80 micrograms, after 18 hours the body would have gotten rid of 40 micrograms. Of the 40 micrograms remaining after 18 more hours had passed (total of 36 hours) 20 micrograms more would be lost leaving 20 micrograms. This goes on until all of the mercury has been dissipated.

It is possible, depending upon the amount of mercury contained in the food we eat or in the air we breathe, to have some detectable level of mercury in our expired breath. However, there is one final point I would like to make on this subject. It is extremely noble for the Councils to be concerned about our potential body burden of mercury that may be derived from food and other sources. IT HAS ABSOLUTELY NOTHING TO DO WITH DETERMINING THE SAFETY OF DENTAL AMALGAM.

ARGUMENT 4
THERE IS NO SCIENTIFIC EVIDENCE TO INDICATE THAT INHALING VERY SMALL DOSES OF MERCURY INCREASE THE INCIDENCE OF DISEASE OR CAUSE HIGHER MORTALITY RATES IN ANYONE INCLUDING DENTAL PERSONNEL WHO HAVE A MUCH GREATER EXPOSURE

SOURCE: JADA, Vol 106, April 1983.
TITLE: Safety of Dental Amalgam.
AUTHOR: Council on Dental Materials, Instruments and Equipment
Council on Dental Therapeutics.
STATEMENT: "Reinhardt et al (2) reported evidence of mercury vapor expired after restorative treatment. Mercury levels in expired air during removal of amalgam ranged from 160 ng/min to less than 40 ng/min and the level following amalgam replacement is about 10 ng/min for up to 200 minutes. No further measurement was made after this period. There is no recorded scientific evidence, of mercury vapor toxicity resulting from this level (10 ng/min) of mercury vapor. Further, none of these measured amounts of released mercury vapor have been documented as being associated with various diseases and/or medical conditions. Furthermore and it is most significant to note that there is no documented scientific evidence to suggest that dentists and dental office personnel who are exposed to much greater amounts of mercury vapor have a greater incidence of certain medical conditions or higher mortality rates as compared to the general population." (the terminology of ng/min means nanograms per minute and represents one billionth of a gram of elemental mercury. Each .100 milligram per cubic meter equals 12.5 nanograms of elemental mercury for each 10 second count).
FOR: Two references are cited in this portion of the ADA policy statement. The first is the work of Dr. Reinhardt and his associates who published in 1979 the preliminary findings of their research which involved the measurement of mercury vapor in expired breath after restorative treatment. The second reference refers to a study titled *"Mortality of Dentists, 1968 to 1972"* which was done by the Bureau of Economic Research and Sta-

tistics of the ADA and published in the JADA, Vol 90, January 1975. Both are excellent studies.

AGAINST: The ADA references the work of Dr. Reinhardt and his associates as proof of their position that the mercury vapor released from amalgam fillings is only a temporary phenomenon, and that the temporary detectable level is so low that it could not possibly contribute to or cause any problems with our health.

In a sense, the ADA is comparing apples and oranges and would have us believe that they are both the same. Dr. Reinhardt's work deals with determining the level of mercury vapor present during the process of removing and replacing an amalgam filling in a tooth. The purpose behind the experiment was to determine if procedures used by the dentist in performing work could minimize the patient's exposure to mercury vapor. The experiments were also intended to determine the length of time increased levels of mercury vapor would be present in the patient's breath after the work had been completed.

Dr. Reinhardt, in discussing his results, and those of his colleagues, states "The levels of mercury recorded in this study are low and quite transient. Consequently this study agrees with Frykholm's conclusion that mercury exposure occurring from the removal or insertion of amalgam restorations will not give rise to systemic mercury poisoning in dental patients." The paper concludes with the following sentence: "The significance of repeated exposure to small amounts of mercury vapor is not entirely understood, but consideration should be given to techniques that minimize exposure to both patients and dental personnel."

More importantly, Dr. Reinhardt states: "Statistical analysis was directed toward determining whether there was a difference between the amount of mercury vapor expired before and after the restorative procedure." What that statement means is that detectable levels of mercury were measured in the patients' mouths before anything was done and that this level only increased very slightly 200 minutes after the procedure of removing and installing a new amalgam filling had been completed. Citing Dr. Reinhardt's work immediately following Dr. Svares experiments in which he and his colleagues measured the expired breath of patients before and after chewing gum, leads the reader to the conclusion that they need not be very concerned with the results of Dr. Svare's work. Nothing could be further from the truth.

The results of the experiments related to mercury vapor levels after chewing were very dramatic. The work of Dr. Svare's group which was outlined in Argument 3 concludes with this statement: "It is thereby concluded that the possibility for significant mercury vapor exposure from dental amalgam in humans exists."

This leads us to the very positive statements made by the ADA concerning the lack of any scientific proof that low levels of mercury vapor from amalgam fillings are associated with any diseases or medical conditions and that mortality rates of dental personnel are no different that of the general population.

The key of course to the first part of the position is the phrase "scientific proof". This puts us face to face with the rigid scientific doctrine that precludes acceptance of "anecdotal" evidence as scientific proof. For example, you might have 500 cases on file that demonstrate that a particular disease or medical condition alleviated or was cured upon removal of amalgam fillings and their replacement with a non-metal composite. This could not be considered as valid scientific proof. What you would have to do to satisfy the scientific proof criteria is take those same 500 people, who had been helped by removal of their amalgam fillings, and put the amalgam fillings back into their teeth to see if the same disease or medical condition reappeared. Even with that, the results might be questioned because of psychological coniserations where it is possible to have a person get better or sicker by suggestion only.

This brings us to the heart of the problem which is dose-response relationships. How much of any poison or toxic substance must an individual take or what degree of exposure must the individual be subjected to before some clinical, identifiable symptom or sign develops? Consequently, it would be a straightforward experiment to take separate groups of animals and subject them to different levels of mercury vapor and record the resulting signs and symptoms. The animals could then be killed and dissected and the experiment would have shown what symptoms or signs the animals displayed at certain dose levels and what internal damage may have been done to cells, organs, glands, or body fluids. What experiments of this type cannot show is how much damage might occur from very small exposures over a period of years.

It is important that you fully understand the significance of this dose-response relationship. There are literally hundreds of scientific papers that show mercury can effect and cause some detectable damage to almost every component of the human body or comparable component of an animal body. However, there does not seem to be any way of proving or demonstrating in a human body that mercury is the sole cause of the detectable damage. To prove this in humans, we would have to be maintained in a totally sterile environment and not subjected to any other known toxic substance except mercury. This of course, is impossible. We are subjected to thousands of chemicals and pollutants in the course of our lifetime simply from the routine acts of eating and breathing.

Consequently it appears that for anyone to make categorical statements that there is absolutely no danger from mercury in amalgam fillings, they would have to compare apples to apples. By this I mean that you simply cannot lump the entire population into one grouping for any type of statistical analysis. To be correct, you would have to analyze that segment of the population who had no amalgam fillings as one group and analyze the remaining group with amalgam fillings as another segment of the population. To my knowledge, such studies have never been done.

When the ADA makes a positive statement that dental personnel have the same incidence of certain medical conditions and mortality rates as compared to the general population, it is a true statement of the facts available from existing data. What is not stated is the fact that like most of the general population to which it is being compared, most dentists have amalgam fillings in their mouths. Therefore should there by any statistical difference? The study cited by the ADA to support their statement on the comparability of dental personnel to the rest of the population, was only done on dentists. There have been no in depth studies done on diseases, medical conditions or mortality on any other personnel working in the dental office, that I have been able to find. Accordingly, I cannot understand how the ADA can make a positive statement concerning this segment of dental personnel. It is the dental assistants, who handle and mix the amalgam, that should really be studied, as that is when the greatest degree of exposure occurs.

What is required, at this point in our evolution, are epidemiological and mortality studies that will portray the incidence of specific diseases or the cause of death under three major sub-divisions of the population: those with amalgam fillings, those who have never had amalgam fillings, and those who have appliances or other devices installed that contain dissimilar metals. The results of such studies may well provide clues to many of the disease states or medical conditions which are presently identified as emanating from an unknown cause.

ARGUMENT 5
MEASUREMENT OF MERCURY CONTENT OF THE URINE IS A RELIABLE INDICATOR OF WHETHER AN INDIVIDUAL MAY SUFFER ANY BIOLOGICAL EFFECTS FROM EXPOSURE TO MERCURY

SOURCE: JADA, Vol 106, April 1983
TITLE: Safety of Dental Amalgams.
AUTHORS: Council on Dental Materials, Equipment and Instruments
               Council on Dental Therapeutics
STATEMENT: "Studies, using radioactive mercury in amalgam restorations, have shown that the urinary excretion of tagged mercury increased 2.5 ug/1 on the 5th day after insertion of an amalgam restoration, and decreased to zero after seven or eight days. On removal of the restorations, the level of tagged mercury in urine increased to 5 ug/1 and then dropped to zero in two days. (4) Studies in humans (5–7) have repeatedly demonstrated and documented that biological effects, particularly central nervous system effects, are not manifested by the most sensitive neurological measurements until the human urinary mercury level reaches 500 ug/1. This level is 170 times the average urinary mercury excretion (3 ug/1) of the general public." NOTE:

The term ug/1 is scientific notation expressing micrograms per liter.

FOR: The ADA has cited four references to support their statement. The first (footnote 4) references the work of Dr. K. O. Frykholm which was a comprehensive study published as a separate issue supplement to the Swedish Journal, Acta Odontologica Scandinavica, Volume 15, 1957. Footnotes 5 and 6 refer to studies done by Langolf and his associates that were published in 1978 and 1979. Footnote 7 references a study by Miller and his associates published in 1975.

In Dr. Frykholm's study, silver amalgam containing radioactive mercury was inserted in the teeth of 5 male volunteer patients. After 7 days, the radioactive amalgam was removed and replaced with regular amalgam. The urine and feces excreted in 24 hours was collected every day during the 7 days the radioactive fillings were in place and for 7 days afterwards. Both the urine and feces were analyzed for mercury utilizing a Scintillation counter. The Langolf, et al. studies were to determine whether existing occupational hygiene controls were adequate to prevent neurotoxic effects in workers exposed to heavy metals, solvents and pesticides. The studies were done over a 6 year period. The researchers set up a series of tests for mercury exposed groups that measured the neurological functions of tremor, psychomotor performance, memory function, and nerve conduction. Each worker's level of mercury exposure was estimated by doing a monthly analysis of the amount of mercury in samples of their urine. A control level of 500 micrograms per liter of urine was established. Their results did indicate that if there were more than 500 micrograms of mercury present in the urine, the workers exhibited detectable changes in neuromuscular tremor power and in tremor frequency. However this level was not found to correlate well with short term memory loss. The work of Miller and his associates was similar in nature although they did not focus on specific urine mercury levels.

AGAINST: There has been a tremendous amount of controversy concerning the use of mercury urine levels as the diagnostic basis for determining toxic effects of exposure to mercury. I believe Goldwater and his associates said it best in their article published in 1964, "Mercury in the urine can no longer influence the living organism, since it has left the body. What it may have done in the course of its absorption, transport, metabolism and excretion is far more important." I think this really gets to the heart of the overall problem concerning the use of amalgam as a filling material. Don't tell me how much mercury my body is getting rid of. Tell me how much is still in my body, where it is, and what it is doing to me.

The controversy rages on even today although through the years there has been a great accumulation of scientific research that concludes that urinary levels of mercury have little or no diagnostic value: Fleishman, 1928; Goldwater, 1957; Noe, 1960; Meyer, 1961; Jacobs et al, 1964; Report of an International Committee: Maximum allowable concentrations of mercury, 1969; Siedlecki, 1971; Hibbard and Smith, 1972; Wallach, 1972; Cutright, 1973; Shofer, 1974; Eastmond and Holt, 1975; Yamaguchi et al, 1977, just to name a few.

From the technical standpoint, the procedures and instruments utilized for mercury analysis have undergone major changes over the years. The problem was considered critical enough that in 1978, the National Academy of Sciences published a comprehensive work titled "An Assessment of Mercury in the Environment" in which they included a 27 page Appendix on Mercury Analytical Methods. One of the points brought out in the Appendix is "Techniques for trace metal analyses have undergone considerable improvement in the past 10 years, leading to a need for assessment of earlier analyses." Another major point made was that unless the sample was "fixed" with certain acids, and stored in a proper container the loss of mercury from the sample to be analyzed could be significant. For example approximately 50% of the mercury in the sample could be lost in 1.5 days if proper procedures are not followed.

Scientists are continually discovering new factors that affect the amount of mercury that is excreted in the urine under various conditions of exposure. For example, Dr. Lie, et al. in 1982, showed that women had a higher mercury urine level than men and that in both sexes there was a reduction in urine mercury with increased age. Kristensen and Hansen in 1980 found that urinary mercury excretion patterns were greatly influenced by selenium levels. Other researchers have also shown that the amino acid cysteine has a bearing on mercury urine levels. I am sure there are many other constituents of our normal food intake that have either a negative or positive effect on our mercury excretion rates. Perhaps the National Acadamy of Sciences puts it in a better perspective when they state: "However, it should be emphasized that the current clinical limits for detecting the effects of methymercury in human populations should not be equated with threshold levels because other more subtle effects, such as behavioral or intellectual deficits, may not be detectable by the clinical procedures that were used." If you would like further proof as to the complexity of this problem, Cherian, et al. in a 1978 paper concluded that "urinary values are more likely to reflect kidney content of mercury".

In Dr. Frykholm's study cited by the ADA, there are some significant aspects that I feel should be pointed out. The first is that there was no evaluation of how much of the radioactive mercury (the amount originally placed in the tooth) was excreted and how much was retained in the body. In the study published by Dr. Cherian and his associates in 1978, which utilized radioactive mercury vapor, they indicate that it is very probable that radioactive mercury is exchanged with a substantial pool of non-radioactive mercury before entering the urine and that the probable location of this pool is the kidneys since the kidneys are the major organs of mercury accumulation in the body. They conclude their article by stating "we therefore have no satisfactory indicator media at this time to indicate brain concentrations of mercury vapor. A similar conclusion has been obtained from animal studies."

Another aspect of Dr. Frykholm's study that is quite significant is that the radioactive fillings were only in place for seven days and, although the radioactive mercury urine levels decreased to zero values on the seventh to eighth day, radioactive mercury was still being detected in the feces of the test patients until the 13th day. This tends to graphically illustrate that the transport and distribution of mercury in the human body is indeed a very complex matter, and critically involves it's biological half-life. In this regard, the material used in Dr. Frykholm's study had a half-life of 47 days. This should have taken over 141 days for the test patients to get rid of all the mercury inhaled during the test.

To insure that you fully understand the significance of this in relation to the overall problem of mercury vapor being released from amalgam fillings, the work of Cherian and his associates showed that the total cumulative amount of radioactive mercury contained in the urine and fecal excretion of their test patients amounted to approximately 11.6% of the retained dose. In this same context, Goodman and Gilman in their book, The Pharmacological Basis of Therapeutics, 6th edition 1980, also state: "Excretion of methylmercury in man is mainly in the feces; less than 10% of a dose appears in urine (Echman et al 1968). The biological half-life of methylmercury in man is about 65 days (Eckman et al, 1968; Bakir et al, 1973)." To make the problem more complex, Clarkson in 1972, in discussing an experiment that had been conducted on rats stated: "These findings suggest that rats exposed daily to mercury would gradually accumulate the metal throughout their life spans." Please bear the last point in mind at all times because I think what the research I have quoted says, is that all of the mercury doesn't come out of our bodies and that as long as we have a continuous source, our bodies will continue to accumulate mercury in almost every organ over our entire life span.

With regard to the work of Langolf et al, they are addressing an industrial exposure problem involving concentrations of mercury vapor in the work place. I cannot really take exception to their findings that there is a relationship between urine mercury levels greater than 500 micrograms per liter and manifestations of neurological damage.

However, not stated by the ADA, is another finding of the Langolf group which I consider to be more significant to the problem we all are concerned with. The results of their testing of short term memory showed a decrease in short term memory capacity and that these sub-clinical short term memory effects could occur at urinary mercury levels maintained consistently below the 500 microgram limit. They also concluded that these short term memory changes resemble those that occur with aging and state "In fact, the changes in memory function associated with an increase in twelve month average urinary mercury of only 100 micrograms per liter may be functionally comparable to the effects of 10 years of aging.''

Based on a comprehensive review of the literature, the prevailing view of most scientists and researchers is that the use of mercury urine levels as a valid and reliable indicator of potential damage to the human body is without merit. Future research efforts must concentrate on determining what damage is being done to our bodies by the mercury that isn't excreted in our urine, feces, breath or sweat, or in the milk of nursing mothers.

ARGUMENT 6
ONLY INDIVIDUALS SENSITIVE TO MERCURY SHOULD CONSIDER REPLACING THEIR AMALGAM FILLINGS

SOURCE: JADA, Vol 106, April 1983.
TITLE: Safety of Dental Amalgam.
AUTHOR: Council on Dental Materials, Instruments and Equipment
               Council on Dental Therapeutics
STATEMENT: Two different statements are made. One in the body of the article and the other as the concluding paragraph. "The Association has previously cautioned that in extremely rare cases, individuals may develop either mercury sensitivity or an allergic reaction from contact with mercury. Patients, as well as dental office personnel, may be affected. Symptoms may vary from a local dermatitis near recently placed amalgam restorations to a generalized erythema over the entire body.'' (Dermatitis is defined as an inflammation of the skin. Erythema is defined as a flush or redness of the skin produced by congestion of the capillaries) "The Association wishes to emphasize that, except in an individual sensitive to mercury, there is no reason why a patient should seek at this time to have amalgam restorations (silver fillings) removed. Indeed, the effect of such a procedure and further restorative operations could be detrimental to the patient's oral health, including the unnecessary loss of teeth, and cannot be justified.''
FOR: The ADA cites no scientific studies or references to support their position.
AGAINST: The simple act of reading those statements leaves

one with the impression that except for a very few individuals in the world, amalgam is completely safe. Chapter 7 of this book addresses the pathology or biological changes in the human body attributable to mercury toxicity so I won't address them at this time.

It is important to explore the subject of sensitivity and allergy to mercury. Dorland's Illustrated Medical Dictionary defines sensitivity as "the state or quality of being sensitive; often used to denote a state of abnormal responsiveness to stimulation, or of responding quickly and acutely"; and defines allergy as "a hypersensitive state acquired through exposure to a particular allergen, re-exposure bringing to light an altered capacity to react. Originally, the term denoted any altered reactivity, whether decreased or increased, but is now usually used to denote a hypersensitive state. Allergies may be classified as immediate and delayed." Dorland's goes on to define 21 different categories of allergies.

Of the 21 categories of allergy defined, we should be concerned with three of them in regard to amalgam fillings. The first is CONTACT ALLERGY, "hypersensitiveness marked by an eczematous reaction to contact between the epidermis and the allergen" (epidermis is the skin and eczematous means an inflammation of the skin that is usually identified by redness, itching, small bumps or elevations, weeping, oozing and crusting). The second category is DELAYED ALLERGY, "an allergic response which appears hours or days after application or absorption of an allergen; it includes contact dermatitis and bacterial allergy." The last category is LATENT ALLERGY, "allergy which is not manifested by symptoms but which may be detected by tests."

Based on the definitions, it doesn't appear that there would be much difference between sensitive or allergic. Both would provoke some type of reaction. What I don't understand is how the ADA can imply that there can be any reaction at all from contact with mercury once the amalgam is installed in a tooth. That is because in a special article printed in the American Dental Association News, dated January 2, 1984, the Association makes the following statement "When mercury is combined with metals used in dental amalgam, its toxic properties are made harmless." If that statement is true then I suppose we should consider mercury in the same category as some of the common foods we get allergies to such as milk, wheat and eggs. To do that though we would have to get the "harmless mercury" into our bodies some way. This begins to sound more like a good mystery novel plot because the ADA also maintains that the mercury doesn't come out of the amalgam filling. So how can we develop allergies to it????

If I were a dentist, I would be very concerned about what the Association has said in their policy statement. They have placed the burden of identifying which patients may be sensitive or allergic directly on the dentist *without providing any guidelines* or tests on how to identify them.

A search of the literature revealed that some of the first symptoms related to oral health that the body displays in reacting to mercury are: bleeding gums, loss of bone (loose teeth), metallic taste in the mouth, and foul breath. How many of you have ever had one or more of these symptoms, and gone to your dentist and had him, or her, say "It looks like you might be sensitive to the mercury in your amalgam fillings"? Instead we are usually given a pretty good dose of "guilt" therapy by the dentist inferring that it is all our fault because we haven't brushed properly, flossed properly, or eaten the proper foods, etc. etc. Those reasons may all be true, but it could also be very probable that we are having a reaction to the mercury in the amalgam fillings. An allergic reaction, which the ADA dismisses by simply having a policy that states "allergic reactions are extremely rare". Nowhere do they have anything published that tells the dentist if he observes such symptoms he should actively consider investigating the possibility that the patient may be having an allergic reaction to mercury or the amalgam itself or possibly one of the other metals in the amalgam. This in spite of the fact that there are evaluation methods, equipment, and tests available to assist the dentist in determining whether a patient may be allergic.

Throughout the documented history of medical and dental use of mercury there has been published evidence attesting to its potency as an allergen. In some few cases, the severity of the reaction has resulted in death. This is not intended to be a scare statement on my part, but merely a statement of fact. It is truly tragic that such events have occurred. My concern is with the fact that mercury is capable of provoking many serious reactions in the human body and that the established agencies, both governmental and private, have not seen fit to do serious research on the subject.

It is true that the ADA has published some research on this subject. One such article was published in the JADA, Vol 92, 1976. This study, done at the University of Texas Dental Branch at Houston, utilized dental students as test subjects and covered the time period from their entry as freshmen until graduation. There were 98 students starting the tests and 74 participants at the end of the test. The students were tested for a CONTACT allergic reaction by means of a patch test. The patch test involved placing a mixture of mercuric chloride and lanolin on a patch that was taped to the student's forearm and left in place for 48 hours. It was checked after 24 hours and the final diagnosis was made at the end of 48 hours when the patch was removed. At that time, a diagnosis was made as to whether or not there was a contact dermatitis reaction. If there was, it was classified as a positive reaction. In their freshman year, 5.2% of the volunteer students had a positive reaction. In their senior year, 10.8% had positive reactions. (It should be pointed out that these were dental students who, in the course of their studies were exposed to the procedure of mixing amalgam and had from 10 exposures in their freshman year to a cumulative total of 54 exposures in their senior year).

I must reemphasize the fact that only a diagnosis of contact allergy was made. No effort was made, nor was the testing protocol designed to determine, if any delayed or latent allergy occurred other than the skin manifestations under the patch. The important words in the definition of delayed allergy are "absorption of an allergen". In other words, we have no way of knowing if the students experienced any physical symptoms such as changes in blood pressure, pulse rate, heart rhythm, etc., because none of the participants were evaluated for these kinds of reactions. It is safe to assume that some of the mercuric chloride entered the body through the skin under the patch as this is a documented avenue of absorption. In fact, the latest technique utilized by the medical profession to administer some drugs is done in almost the same manner, ie. absorbed through the skin from a patch containing the drug which is placed on the skin.

Another finding of the researchers Drs. White and Brandt, who conducted the study, was that there was a discernable relationship in the number of positive reactions of the participants that were related to the age of the fillings. Only 3.8% of the students whose amalgam fillings had been in place five years or less tested positive whereas 6% of those whose amalgam fillings were more than five years old tested positive.

There had been a previous study, similar in nature, done by Djerassi and Berova in Sophia, Bulgaria which was published in the International Dental Journal in 1969. This study did not use dental students as test subjects. In fact, anyone who had been in contact with amalgam professionally was specifically excluded from participating in the study. The purpose of their study was to determine: "Whether it is possible that the sensitization from amalgam may be due exclusively to dental restorations; whether the time the amalgam restorations remain in the mouth plays an important part in the manifestation of the allergic reaction; which component of the amalgam plays the leading role in the allergic reaction; which of the factors such as age, sex, occupation, etc. of the patient favor sensitization by amalgam".

The study had 240 test subjects. Of this number, 180 had amalgam fillings and 60 had no amalgam restorations at all. The subjects were divided into 4 groups of 60 persons each according to the following categories:

1. Healthy; with amalgam restorations.
2. Sick (non-allergic diseases); with amalgam restorations.
3. Allergic patients; with amalgam restorations.
4. A control group; without amalgam restorations.

The subjects were then patch tested for allergic reactions not only to mercury, but to the amalgam itself, and each one of its component metals of silver, copper, tin and zinc. These results were read 24 and 48 hours after testing. Their results were much more startling than Drs. White and Brandt's results: 16.1% of the entire group of 180 people with amalgam fillings, exhibited a positive reaction to amalgam and its components. The positive reactions occurred within the groups as follows: 8.3% in healthy persons; 13.3% in non-allergic patients, and 26.6% in allergic patients. Exceptionally significant was the fact that THERE WERE NO POSITIVE REACTIONS IN THE CONTROL GROUP WHO HAD NO AMALGAM FILLINGS. Another major finding that differed significantly from the results of Drs. White and Brandt was the percentage of positive reactions in people with aged fillings: 5.8% in people with restorations less than 5 years old; and 22.52% in people with restorations that were older than 5 years. Another finding of great significance was the number of people who tested positive to the components of amalgam. These results were as follows:

Amalgam—16.1%

Mercury—11%

Copper—6%

Zinc—4%

Silver—3%

Tin—0%

Based on the overall results of their study the authors advanced the hypothesis that "Amalgam can cause the formation of several kinds of antibodies directed to the amalgam complex as a whole, as well as their individual components."

Why were the results of Djerassi and Berova's study ignored by the United States? At the very least, the study should have been duplicated in this country to confirm or deny the results. The fact that test participants without any amalgam fillings did not have any positive reactions should have been reason enough. In regard to the last point, I invite the ADA to tell me how the 60 people in the test did not have any reaction to mercury when they maintain that we get as much mercury out of our food as we could ever get from amalgam fillings!

Do you realize how many people we are talking about that may be having undiagnosed reactions to mercury amalgam in their teeth? There are no statistics that I have been able to find that indicate what percentage of the U.S. population have amalgam fillings in their teeth. For our example here let's be conservative and say 65%, (It is more probably 85 or 90%) and for a total population figure lets only use 200 million. Of that number 130 million (65%) would then have amalgam fillings. If we use the lowest figure from Drs. White and Brandt's study which was

2%, we would have a total of 2,600,000 people who could be allergic to mercury. If we use Djerassi and Berova's findings of 16.1%, there would be 20,930,000 people who could be allergic to the amalgam fillings in their teeth. Is that a significant number? The U.S. Center for Disease Control would consider that a National Epidemic requiring all available resources of the government to be marshalled to find a solution to the problem.

Although I'm not from Missouri, their "show me" attitude seems appropriate for the problem. It would appear to be a prudent action at this time for the National Institutes of Health through their Allergy and Dental Research divisions to set up a test protocol that would answer the question once and for all. That doesn't seem to be too unreasonable a request, especially when you consider some of the grants that have been made to study some really diverse subjects that serve no apparent useful purpose to mankind.

ARGUMENT 7
ONCE MERCURY IS COMBINED WITH OTHER METALS USED IN DENTAL AMALGAM ITS TOXIC PROPERTIES ARE MADE HARMLESS

SOURCE: American Dental Association News, Jan 2, 1984
TITLE: To the Dental Patient.
AUTHOR: American Dental Association.
STATEMENT: "Isn't mercury a poison? When mercury is combined with the metals used in dental amalgam, its toxic properties are made harmless. Moreover, the safety of dental amalgam has been studied for nearly a century, and all documented research indicates that, for the vast majority of dental patients, mercury-containing amalgams present no health hazard."
FOR: This statement is part of a fact sheet prepared by the ADA for dentists to give to any patient who questions the safety of dental amalgam. As the fact sheet was produced for general public consumption, no scientific references were given.
AGAINST: The statement is such a distortion of the truth that I was seriously tempted not to comment on it. However, to not do so would give the statement credibility, of which it has none. Here again, I can only conclude that the ADA is relying heavily

on the work of Dr. Frykholm as the basis of their statement, although I have no proof of that fact. In response to their statement, I challenge the ADA to provide documented scientific proof that even remotely provides any evidence in support of their claim.

Because the statement is taken out of context, and in all fairness to the ADA, I believe everyone reading this book should have the benefit of reading the fact sheet and accompanying editorial.

EDITORIAL

"The American Dental Association has been receiving an increasing number of inquiries from the media concerning the safety of mercury in dental amalgam. Subsequent information provided by our media reporting services tells us that these inquiries are being turned into news stories. Further, the geographical diversity of the news stories suggests that the safety of dental amalgam has become a nationwide issue.

Despite some sensationalized claims in the media that mercury in amalgam has caused a variety of maladies, no one has yet presented credible scientific evidence that properly placed amalgam restorations have been the cause of bodily disorders. In fact, the Association's Council on Dental Materials, Instruments, and Equipment recommends against removing sound restorations.

Still the media coverage may cause concern among your patients over amalgam restorations.

To help you provide accurate information to your patients on this issue, the ADA has prepared a fact sheet that appears below. We suggest that you cut it out and reproduce it for distribution for those patients who express concern.

If you don't need it now, keep it on file. You may need it later.

TO THE DENTAL PATIENT

Recent reports in the public media have raised questions as to the safety of dental amalgam. In order to provide you with accurate information on the use and safety of dental amalgam, the American Dental Association has prepared the following answers to the most commonly asked questions about dental amalgam.

WHAT IS DENTAL AMALGAM?

Dental amalgam is the material most often used to fill cavities caused by tooth decay. In general, one or more metals are combined with mercury to form a pliable mass. This material is then condensed in the cavity, which the dentist has cleared of decay. There, it hardens into a dental restoration or filling.

WHICH METALS ARE USED IN DENTAL AMALGAM?

Silver, copper, and tin are the metals commonly used in dental amalgam, sometimes in combination with zinc. Dental amalgam is used in about 75% of all single-tooth fillings.

DOES THE ADA HAVE AN ACCEPTANCE PROGRAM FOR DENTAL AMALGAMS?

Yes. To help dentists choose from among the various brands of dental amalgam on the market, the ADA has established an acceptance program to examine these products for safety and effectiveness. To date, more than 100 brands of dental amalgam have been accepted for the dentist's use.

WHY IS MERCURY USED IN DENTAL AMALGAM?

When combined with silver or other metals, the mercury produces a chemical reaction that causes the filling to harden after it has been placed in the cavity.

IS THIS SOMETHING NEW?

No. the basic technique has been used to restore decayed teeth for about 150 years.

ISN'T MERCURY A POISON?

When mercury is combined with the metals used in dental amalgam, its toxic properties are made harmless. Moreover, the safety of dental amalgam has been studied for nearly a century, and all documented research indicates that, for the vast majority of dental patients, mercury-containing amalgams present no health hazard. Mercury in small quantities is found naturally in the human system. And the average mercury level found in the general public is more than 100 times lower than the level at which harmful effects are usually reported.

AREN'T SOME PEOPLE ALLERGIC TO MERCURY?

In rare cases, a patient may experience an allergic reaction to mercury, usually in the form of dermatitis or skin rash. To guard against this very remote possibility, the ADA recommends that dentists maintain a complete medical history for each patient. If the patient is known to have such an allergy, the dentist may choose some other restorative material, something other than dental amalgam.

WHAT OTHER FILLING MATERIALS ARE AVAILABLE?

Gold is often used to fill teeth, either in pure form or alloyed with some metal or element other than mercury. Some manufacturers are working to produce composite resins (plastics), which soon may be available as acceptable alternatives to dental amalgam. To date, however, these materials have not proved durable enough to withstand the great pressure generated by chewing. Dental researchers are constantly seeking safe, new methods for restoring decayed teeth. For most patients, though, dental amalgam remains a safe and effective material for filling cavities.

WHAT IS THE "LIFE SPAN" OF A DENTAL AMALGAM?

On the average, amalgams serve for at least ten years, and very often they last considerably longer. Conditions in the mouth are constantly changing, and these changes affect dental materials and their function. Your fillings will last longer if you follow proper procedures for home care and receive regular dental checkups.

American Dental Association
211 East Chicago Avenue
Chicago, Illinois 60611

In closing the argument section of this book, I feel compelled to present further information regarding Dr. Frykholm's work not previously discussed. This is because I believe that his work must be considered as the greatest single factor contributing to the controversy we are confronted with today.

It is unfortunate for the population at large, that his testing protocol was designed as it was and that the better instrumentation and additional knowledge of urine testing subsequently available was not in place when Dr. Frykholm performed his experiments. His work, published in 1957, has been continuously cited since that time by every proponent of continued use of mercury amalgam as a dental restoration material. In effect, because no one seriously questioned his work, the findings of this one researcher have until recently contributed significantly to holding back progress, thereby, curtailing a concerted effort to find acceptable alternative dental filling materials. Why would any individual or corporation expend huge sums of money in research to develop a product to replace something that had been in use for 125 years, was considered safe, was easy to use, and above all was inexpensive.

The basis of Dr. Frykholm's experiments was to determine the extent of exposure to mercury vapor during dental treatment, both to the patient as well as dental personnel. This particular problem was selected because a review of the literature indicated such a study had not previously been done.

Some aspects of his study not discussed in previous arguments in this chapter are included now.

ABSORPTION FROM INHALED AIR: Eight human subjects were utilized and three to four amalgam fillings were to be installed in each patients mouth. Using a General Electric Instantaneous Mercury Vapor Detector, mercury content of the air within the mouth, over the fillings, near the mouths of the dentist and his assistant and in the room itself, was determined at one minute intervals. All of the test patients had previous amalgam fillings that were at least one year old. The results of this phase of the experiment can be summarized as: "Yes", some mercury vapor was present before the new fillings were installed, but this was around zero; and "Yes", the mercury vapor concentration increased during the installation of the amalgam filling. However, after rinsing the mouth and when the restorations had been covered with saliva, the recorded values were close to the ones recorded before the treatment began. Dr. Frykholm concludes this phase by stating that theoretically the most that exposed subjects, among those studied, could have taken up was about 0.1 milligram of mercury by inhalation and that this amount is far from sufficient to make the mercury up-take injurious.

Another aspect of this phase that seems totally unsatisfactory, is that no measurements were made after chewing and that the temperature measurements in the room were only 68 degrees Fahrenheit and the temperature in the patient's mouth was only 89.6 degrees Fahrenheit. Since mercury is more volatile with increased temperature and compression stress, it would seem reasonable to assume that a normal body temperature of 98.6 degrees Fahrenheit and the stress and frictional heat of chewing should have been considered as an essential part of the protocol. The latter statement is made with full knowledge and appreciation of the fact that Dr. Frykholm was only attempting to determine exposures during installation of new fillings.

There also has to be a question raised concerning the limitations of the measuring instrument used which could not detect mercury vapor levels that were lower than 10 micrograms and which used a 2 second sampling for the evaluation. The instruments available today read mercury vapor levels as low as 1 microgram based on a 10 second exposure sampling.

Perhaps the most important aspect of this experiment is the statement that the levels of mercury vapor encountered could not possibly be considered injurious. That is a subjective judgment without scientific substantiation as no pathological evaluations were done and any previously published literature providing indications to the contrary were simply dismissed or merely mentioned in passing.

Some of the authors quoted by Frykholm who had published papers indicating a significant danger from mercury released from amalgam fillings were: Professor Stock in 1926, with subsequent articles through 1939; Toverud in 1932; Steffensen in 1934; and Hadenque in 1950. Publications after Dr. Frykholm's article was published in 1957 that have indicated findings and conclusions contrary to his were: Dr. Svare, et al. in 1980 who concluded their article with the statement "that the possibility for significant vapor exposure from dental amalgam exists"; Beste and Zoller in an article published in Dental Student, April 1976, stated that "elemental mercury vapor, in its final distribution, is found concentrated in the brain at levels 10 times those found elsewhere in the body."; and Bauer and First in their article published in the California Dental Association Journal, June 1982, state "even at low levels (mercury) can affect the motor control centers of the brain."

SALIVA EFFECTS: This was the 2nd area of experimentation conducted by Dr. Frykholm. There were two distinct aspects addressed. The first concerns the determination of whether saliva coating an amalgam filling stops the release of mercury vapor, and the 2nd deals with whether mercury is soluble in saliva.

The question of whether saliva coats the fillings and stops release of mercury was addressed during his first experiment involving the measurement of mercury vapor after a new amalgam filling had been installed. His statement on this is quoted as follows: "The protective effect of the saliva immediately coating the fillings after the insertion is completed, reduces the further vapor evolution to insignificant amounts." As previously pointed out, there is a serious question regarding the protocol used in arriving at this conclusion.

Contrary to Dr. Frykholm's conclusion the following authors published papers confirming little, if any, protection from release of mercury vapor is gained by a film of saliva over the amalgam: Stock, 1926 and 1939; Trakhtenberg 1969: Gay, et al, 1979; Svare, et al, 1981; Abraham, et al, 1984; and Utt, 1984.

With regard to the question of whether mercury is soluble in saliva, Dr. Frykholm concluded that silver amalgam is only slightly soluble. For you, the reader, the significance of whether mercury is soluble in saliva simply means that if the amalgam filling does release mercury compounds, they would dissolve in your saliva and then be absorbed in the mucous tissues of the mouth and gastrointestinal tract. It appears that here again there is a problem in the basic assumption from which the experiment proceeded. As part of his qualifying remarks relating to the saliva experiments, Dr. Frykholm states "It is well known that a silver amalgam filling which is already hard remains practically unchanged for many years as far as its volume, weight and shape are concerned.". Although the amount of research prior to 1957 appears sketchy, there were two reports that indicated finding mercury in saliva (which would also indicate that mercury compounds were being released from the amalgam filling thereby decreasing its volume and weight), Jensen and Dane in 1954 and Breguet in 1952. Subsequent research totally refutes any idea that a silver amalgam filling remains unchanged for many years.

Researchers have shown that a substantial loss of mercury occurs. This was proven by actually weighing the amalgam fillings in teeth that had been extracted. What these researchers found was an astonishing loss of as high as 84% of the original mercury content of the amalgam filling as shown in the following table:

PERCENT OF MERCURY CONTENT
REMAINING IN OLD FILLINGS

Researcher	Year	% Remaining
Radics	1970	16 to 40%
Gasser	1972	16 to 40%
Gasser	1976	16 to 40%
Hanson	1982	16 to 43%
Pleva	1982	27% Average

What this means to anyone with amalgam fillings in their mouth should be obvious. Depending on the number of fillings in your mouth you could have swallowed or inhaled anywhere from 30 to 560 milligrams of mercury particles or vapor over the years. (Stofen, 1974).

REFERENCES

ARGUMENT 1

1. Safety of Dental Amalgam. Journal of the American Dental Association, Vol 106, pages 519–520, 1983.

2. Bauer, J. G. and First, H. A., The Toxicity of Mercury in Dental Amalgam. California Dental Association Journal, Vol 10, Pages 47–61, 1982.

ARGUMENT 2

1. Berlin, M. H., Nordberg, G. F., and Serenius, F. On the Site and Mechanism of Mercury Vapor Resorption in the Lung. Archives of Environmental Health, Vol 18, pages 42–50, 1969.

2. Kudsk, F. Nielson., Absorption of Mercury from the Respiratory Tract in Man. Acta Pharmacology Toxicology, Vol 23, Pages 250–258, 1965.

3. Clarkson, T. W., The Pharmacology of Mercury Compounds. Annual Review Pharmacology, Vol 12, pages 375–406, 1972.

4. Jernelov, A., Chapter 4, Conversion of Mercury Compounds in: Chemical Fallout, Miller, M. W. and Berg G. C. (Eds) Charles C. Thomas, Springfield Ill., 1969.

5. Abdulla, M., Arnesjo, B., and Ihse, I., Scandinavian Journal of Gastroenterology, Vol 8, page 565, 1973.

6. Edwards, T., and McBride, B. C., Nature (London) Vol 253, page 462, 1975.

7. Rowland, I. R., Grasso, P., and Davies, M. J., The Methylation of Mercuric Chloride by Human Intestinal Bacteria. Experientia, Vol 31, pages 1064–1065, 1975.

8. Heintze, V., Edwardson, S., Derand, R., and Birkhead, D., Methylation of Mercury from Dental Amalgam and Mercuric Chloride by Oral Streptococci In Vitro. Scandanavian Journal of Dental Research, Vol 91, Issue 2, pages 150–152, 1983.

ARGUMENT 3

1. Stofen, D. Dental Amalgam—A Poison In Our Mouth? Toxicology, Vol 2, pages 355–358, 1974.

2. Souder, W. and Sweeney, W. T., Is Mercury Poisonous in Dental Amalgam Restorations? The Dental Cosmos, Vol 73, Issue 12, pages 1145–1152, Dec 1931.

3. Frykholm, K. O., On Mercury From Dental Amalgam: Its Toxic and

Allergic Effects And Some Comments On Occupational Hygiene. Acta Odontologica Scandinavica, Vol 15, Suppl 22, pages 1–123, 1957.

4. Svare, C. W., Peterson, L. C., Reinhardt, J. W., Boyer, D. B., Frank, C. W., Gay, D. D., and Cox, R. D., The Effect of Dental Amalgams on Mercury Levels in Expired Air. Journal of Dental Research, Vol 60, Issue 9, pages 1668–1671, 1981.

5. Hursh, J. B., Clarkson, T. W., Cherian, M. B., Vostal, J., and Vander Mallie, R., Clearance of Mercury (Hg-197, Hg-203) Vapor Inhaled by Human Subjects. Archives Environmental Health, Vol 31, pages 302–309, 1976.

ARGUMENT 4

1. Reinhardt, J. W., Boyer, D. B., Gay, D. D., Cox, R. , Frank, C. W., and Svare, C. W., Mercury Vapor Expired After Restorative Treatment: Preliminary Study. Journal of Dental Research, Vol 58, Issue 1, page 2005, 1979.

ARGUMENT 5

1. Frykholm, K. O., (see No. 3 under Argument 3)

2. Langolf, G. D., et al. Prospective Study of Psychomotor Function and Urinary Mercury of Mercury Cell Chlor-Alkali Plant Workers. Rada. Toksikol Vol 30, page 275, 1979.

3. Langolf G. D., et al. Evaluation of Workers Exposed to Elemental Mercury Rada. Toksikol Vol 30, page 275, 1979.

3. Langolf G. D., et al. Evaluation of Workers Exposed to Elemental Mercury Using Quantitative Test of Tremor and Neuromuscular Function. American Industrial Hygiene Association Journal, Vol 39, page 976, 1978.

4. Miller, J. M., et al. Subclinical Psychomotor and Neuromuscular Changes in Workers Exposed to Inorganic Mercury. American Industrial Hygiene Association Journal, Vol 10, Page 725, 1976.

5. Noe, F. E., Chronic Mercurial Intoxication: A Review. Industrial Medicine and Surgery, Vol 29, pages 559–564, 1960.

6. Eastmond, C. J., and Holt, S., A Case Of Acute Mercury Vapor Poisoning. Postgraduate Medical Journal, Vol 51, pages 428–430, 1975.

7. Wallach, L., Aspiration Of Elemental Mercury: Evidence of Absorption Without Toxicity. New England Journal of Medicine, Vol 287, pages 178–179, 1972.

8. Kristensen, P., and Hansen J. C., Urinary And Fecal Excretion Of Selenium ($Na_2{}^{75}SeO_3$ and Mercury $^{203}HgCl_2$) Administered Separately and Simultaneously to Mice. Toxicology, Vol 16, pages 39–47, 1980.

9. Goldwater, L. J., The Toxicology of Inorganic Mercury. Annals of The New York Academy of Science, Vol 65, Issue 5, 1957.

10. Report Of An International Committee: Maximum Allowable Concentrations Of Mercury Compounds (MAC Values). Archives Environmental Health, Vol 19, pages 891–901, 1969.

11. Jacobs, M. B., Ladd, A. C., and Goldwater, L. J., Absorbtion And Excretion Of Mercury In Man VI Significance Of Mercury In Urine. Archives Environmental Health, Vol 9, pages 454–463, 1964.

12. Cutright, D. E., et al. Systemic Mercury Level Caused By Inhaling Mist During High Speed Grinding. Journal of Oral Medicine, Vol 28, Issue 4, pages 100–104, 1973.

13. National Academy of Science. An Assessment Of Mercury In The Environment. A Report Prepared By The Panel On Mercury Of The Coordinating Committee For Scientific And Technical Assessments Of Environmental Pollutants. National Research Council, National Academy of Science, 1978.

14. Lee, A., Gundersen, N., and Korsgaard, K.J., Mercury In Urine—Sex, Age and Geographic Differences In A Reference Population. Scandinavian Journal Work Environment Health, Vol 8, pages 129–133, 1982.

15. Cherian, M. G., Hursh, J. B., Clarkson, T. W., and Allen J., Radioactive Mercury Distribution In Biological Fluids and Excretion In Human Subjects After Inhalation Of Mercury Vapor. Archives Environmental Health, Vol 33, Issue 3, pages 109–114, 1978.

16. Clarkson, T. W., (See No. 3 of Argument 2)

17. Eckman, L., et al. Metabolism and Retention of Methyl—203—Mercury Nitrate in Man. Nordic Medicine, Vol 79, pages 450–456, 1968.

18. Goodman and Gillman's., The Pharmacological Basis of Therapeutics, 6th Ed, 1980. Macmillan Publishing Co., Inc., New York.

19. Bakir, F., et al. Methylmercury Poisoning in Iraq, An Interuniversity Report. Science, Vol 181, pages 230–241, 1973.

20. Langolf G. D., et al. Measurements of Neurological Functions in Evaluations of Exposure to Neurotoxic Agents. Annals of Occupational Hygiene, Vol 24, Issue 3, pages 293–296, 1981.

ARGUMENT 6

1. Dorland's Illustrated Medical Dictionary, 25th Edition, 1974. W. B. Saunders Co., Philadelphia.

2. White R. R., and Brant, R. L., Development of Mercury Hypersensitivity Among Dental Students. Journal of the American Dental Association, Vol 92, pages 1204–1207, 1976.

3. Djerassi, E., and Berova, N., The Possibilities of Allergic Reactions From Silver Amalgam Restorations. International Dental Journal, Vol 19, Issue 4, pages 481–488, 1969.

ARGUMENT 7

1. Stock, A., The Hazards of Mercury Vapor. Zeitschr Angew Chem, Vol 39, pages 461–488, 1926.

2. Toverud, G. Om "kvikksolvforgiftning" fra amalgam. Den Norske Tannlaegeforenings tidende, Vol 42: pages 181–191, 1932.

3. Steffensen, K., Om kronisk Kviksolvforgiftning foraarsaget af Tand-plomber. Ugeskr. laeger, Vol 96, pages 855–858, 1934.

4. Hadengue, A., et al. Note sur lelimination urinaire du mercure. Arch Mal Profess, Vol 11, pages 45–47, 1950.

5. Jensen, A. T., and Dano, M., Chrystallography of Dental Calculus and the Precipitation of Certain Calcium Phosphates. J Dent Res, Vol 33, pages 741–750, 1954.

6. Breguet, P., Action de la salive sur les amalgames dentaires. These. Geneve, 1952.

7. Abraham, J. E., et al. The effect of dental amalgam restorations on blood mercury. J Dent Res, Vol 63, Issue 1, pages 71–73, Jan 1984.

8. Utt, H. D., "Mercury breath" . . . How much is too much? Cal Dent Assoc J, pages 41–45, February 1984.

CHAPTER 5

DO WE REALLY HAVE ELECTRICITY IN OUR MOUTHS?

The answer is a strong "yes", if we have more than one kind of metal in our mouths. A weak "yes" if only one kind of metal is present. (Phillips, 1973) (Hyams et al, 1933) (Solomon, 1933) The answer is based in chemistry where all metals have been identified or graded by their electropotential. You may think that a piece of metal is a solid object that remains silent and unchanged forever. That is not the case at all. If that were true, then the metal in our cars would never corrode (rust). In chemistry, all metals have been classified by their electropotential from strong to weak. In one sense you might say that all metals are reservoirs of energy which are called electrons. The stronger the energy capability of the metal the more electrons it can attract. The weaker the energy force of the metal the easier it releases or gives up some of its electrons. This is so because electrons are always negative and always move from the weaker to the stronger attraction. Therefore, if you can get these electrons flowing through some kind of a conductor or transport medium, you will have an electrical current.

That last sentence is the key. The stronger energy source has to be connected in some way to the weaker energy source in order to have the electrons flow from one to the other. Aqueous solutions that have metal ions in them are called electrolytes and are capable of conducting or transporting an electrical current.

The aqueous solutions that don't have any metal ions are called nonelectrolytes. SO WHAT? What has all this got to do with me and my mouth?

Your saliva, which is an aqueous solution, is full of metal ions, particularly the life essential ones like sodium, potassium, calcium and magnesium, and also many others. This means that our saliva is an electrolyte. Now we have an electrolyte in our mouths bathing all our teeth and tissues with a film of liquid that has the capability of transporting or conducting electrical current from one point to another.

What else do we have in our mouths? Oxygen, which can cause metal to give up electrons by a process called oxidation (just like on your car when it starts to rust); strong and weak acids from our food and drinks, such as coffee, tea, colas, and citrus juices that can cause a chemical action to occur in the metals; friction caused from chewing which also generates heat; and temperature differences from the hot and cold food and drinks that we ingest. All of these are capable of exciting or generating activity in metal.

Where do we stand when we have metal in our teeth like amalgam, or gold, or chromium, or aluminum, etc.? What we have, is a potential electrical generating plant. Everything that's needed to cause electrons to flow from one point to another is present. We also have tissue composed of millions of cells that all have some of the electrolytes around them or inside of them. We also have nerves which, for our oversimplified description, can act as transmission lines carrying electric charges to other parts of the body.

Let's explore a common example of a gold crown and an amalgam filling next to it and see what can happen. The first thing we have to investigate is corrosion of the amalgam filling. Webster's Dictionary defines corrode as ''1. to eat away gradually as if by gnawing, especially chemical action. 2. to impair or deteriorate.'' When an amalgam filling is installed in a tooth, it is subjected to all the chemicals we put in our mouths which are part of our normal intake of food and drink, and also to some of those produced by our own bodies. The acid or alkaline status of our saliva will vary with our food intake and individual body chemistry. All of this starts corroding or rusting away that amalgam as soon as it is installed. That's one reason why you periodically have to have amalgam fillings replaced. Maybe you have even had the experience of a filling becoming loose and falling out. I wonder how that happened? Although the ADA has stated (ADA News, Jan 2, 1984) that amalgam fillings last for 10 years, this is not a correct statement. Some will of course, but recent research (Smales and Gerke, et al. 1983) has shown that within 3 years, 13% of a group of 720 restorations had heavy surface tarnishing and all 720 already showed some signs of deterioration. Hamilton, et al. 1983, in a 10 year study reported that 35 of 99 amalgam restorations began showing deterioration at the end of the 1st year and that at the end of 10 years only 17% of the original molar restorations remained functional.

Besides the chemical corrosion in our mouths we also have the corrosion that can be caused by the electrical activity we previously discussed. We have both of these factors increasing the corrosion of the amalgam which, in the process, is releasing metal ions into our saliva. This corrosion may also reduce the strength of the filling and cause increased marginal breakdown of the amalgam. There are processes by which mercury (and other metals in the amalgam) is continually being released as vapor and abraded particles.

Let us return to our gold crown and amalgam filling example, and the possible problems (other than the release of mercury) caused by all the electrical activity in our mouths. Electro-galvanic activity associated with having metal in your mouth is not a new discovery or phenomenon. To the best of my knowledge, it was first discussed in scientific literature in 1878 by Dr. Henry S. Chase of St. Louis and Dr. S. B. Palmer of Syracuse N.Y. There have been a tremendous number of studies published since that date, all confirming the electrical discharge phenomonen associated with having metals in our mouths.

Is it significant? To answer that question I would like to quote from a 1933 article by Dr. Hyams and his associates published in the Canadian Medical Association Journal. Please keep in mind that this article was written fifty one (51) years ago:

"Lain, (3) Lippman, (4) Ullman and others have drawn attention to the fact that dissimilar metals in the oral cavity may be responsible for local objective changes such as acute and chronic inflammation, blanched or grayish patches, erosions, ulcers, areas of leukoplakia and pigmentation. Lain has numbered among the objective changes in the metallic dentures, discoloration, areas of erosion, disintegration, loosening of restorations, and maladjustment of dentures. According to him, the complaints which can be due to dissimilar metals in the mouth may include a metallic or salty taste, increased salivary secretion, burning tongue, dryness or tickling sensation in the throat, nerve shocks, nervous irritability and loss of weight. To these we can add, dyspnoea (difficulty in breathing) and diarrhoea. In both patients referred to above the original symptoms could be reproduced by restoring the original local conditions.

Sufficient evidence has now accumulated to indicate definitely that dissimilar metals in the oral cavity can be responsible for local lesions and local and general symptoms. It has been, and can be, shown that electro-galvanic discharges may be present in the oral cavity and the patient remain symptom-free. Perhaps some of the local changes, and, for that matter, general symptoms, can be explained upon a purely chemical basis. Certainly, as Solomon, Reinhardt, and Goodale (5) have shown, there is frequently no direct connection between the amount of current measured and the symptoms present. Recognizing the possibilities suggested by our two cases, it should also be appreciated that dissimilar metals in the mouth which are producing electrogalvanic discharges may be responsible for symptoms even in the absence of a local lesion or changes in the metallic denture present. Perhaps the nature of the patient's diet may be of some moment in such cases. We have tested many substances in solutions. To refer only to a few; when gold and aluminum are combined with milk as the electrolyte a current of 65 microamperes is registered; if an equal quantity of saliva is added to the same combination, 105 microamperes is generated. A weak salt solution under similar conditions registers 400, strong tea 110, zinc chloride mouth wash 300 microamperes.

The treatment is simple. The offending metals present should be replaced. Occasionally, destroying the contact between the dissimilar metal suffices. Before symptoms are attributed to dissimilar metals in the mouth all other important conditions must first be excluded. A milliammeter is inexpensive and easy to handle. Its use in office practice is recommended. It should certainly form part of the equipment of not only dental but also of large medical clinics. Prophylaxis is of course the chief consideration. When dental work is recommended and restorations become necessary, the use of inert metals, preferably noble metals, should always be urged.

If that isn't enough, more recent research has focused on "pain" that may be attributable to this source of electrical discharge. Many researchers have concluded that these electric potentials in the oral cavity may reach 900 millivolts or higher. The number 900 or higher becomes extremely important to us poor mortals when we take a look at the nerves in our bodies and how they transmit impulses to and from one point to another. Those of us outside the medical or scientific community, if asked to, would probably describe a nerve as one long continuous fiber connecting one point to another. We would be totally wrong. A nerve, for our purposes of illustration, can be considered as different lengths of fiber encased in a sheath. At the junction of each length of nerve fiber is a space called a "synapse". To get an impulse across this junction or synapse, it has to be fired electrically. Scientists have shown that the least possible voltage at which an impulse will fire across the synapse on a large nerve is 400 to 450 millivolts. When you think of this in relation to the fact that there are a great number of nerves in our bodies that make their way to the brain through a specific area of our jaws, the problem concerning the point I am making gets much easier to understand.

If a nerve happens to be close enough to a large metal restoration in our mouth that is capable of generating 900 millivolts or more, and the nerve only requires 400 to 450 millivolts to cause it to fire, we have all the ingredients necessary to cause "pain". If the metal in the tooth discharges its electrical current to the nerve, it will cause the nerve to fire and cause a nerve shock which our sensory system will then register as pain (it would be almost the same as sticking a pin or needle into our jaw).

The anatomic pathways pain may take from our upper jaws may explain why some changes can occur in reflexes, emotions, heart and lung functions. These pathways permit the pain to travel the network of nerves of the brain stem right to the hypothalmus and pituitary which are the control centers for our autonomic nervous system and major endocrine glands that produce hormones.

When we probe into repairing decay damage to a tooth by putting a simple amalgam filling in it, we have the potential of opening "Pandora's Box" with regard to the problems that may follow. To adapt President Kennedy's famous quotation to this situation we might well say to our dentist and to the ADA, "Ask not what we patients can do for you, but rather, what can you do for us to solve this problem".

REFERENCES

1. Phillips, R. W., (Editor) Skinner's Science of Dental Materials, 7th Ed, 1973. W. B. Saunders Co., Philadelphia.

2. Solomon, H. A., Reinhard, M. C., and Goodale, H. I., The Possibility of Precancerous Oral Lesions from Electrical Causes. Dental Digest, Vol 39, pages 142–144, April 1933.

3. Smales, R. J., and Gerke, D. C., Three-Year Clinical Evaluation of Four High-Copper Amalgam Alloys, IADR Abstracts, 1983.

4. Hamilton, J. C., et al. Marginal Fracture Not a Predictor of Longevity For Two Dental Amalgam Alloys: A Ten Year Study. Journal of Prosthetic Dentistry, Vol 50, Issue 2, pages 200–202, 1983.

5. Chase, H. S., Some Observations and Experiments Connected with Oral Electricity. American Journal of Dental Science, Vol 12, pages 18–23, 1878–1879.

6. Palmer, S. B., Dental Decay and Filling Materials Considered in Their Electrical Relations. American Journal of Dental Science, Vol 12, pages 105–111, 1878–1879.

7. Hyams, B. L., et al. Dissimilar Metals In The Mouth As A Possible Cause of Otherwise Unexplainable Symptoms. The Canadian Medical Journal, Vol 29, pages 488–491, Nov. 1933.

CHAPTER 6

MERCURY IN MY BODY?
WHERE DOES IT GO?
HOW LONG DOES IT STAY?

This and the following chapters in the book are the most difficult to write about in a form that the general public will be able to understand. The reason for this is that the real information you need to know can only come from highly technical and scientific research articles and books.

These are the real mystery stories of research and what science is all about. The dedication of the men and women who pursue these fields of endeavor make them the true unsung heroes of the the world's war for survival. Although only a few receive the recognition and acclaim they justly deserve. They all deserve and are entitled to our eternal gratitude and respect. Many devote entire lifetimes working to unravel one tiny facet of the greatest mystery in the universe, the human body. Without them, it would not be a very nice world to live in.

Thousands of research papers have been written that either directly or indirectly deal with the toxicity of mercury, and there is no end in sight. Nor should there be, until the scientific community knows, and understands, every nuance about this highly poisonous element. This includes determining exactly what it does in the human body, and perhaps of much more importance, how we can overcome its ill effects and limit future damage from dietary and environmental exposures.

Banning the use of mercury in dentistry and medicine is a

simple way to control some of our exposure. Although science cannot state categorically in all instances that mercury is the sole cause of some symptoms, syndromes or diseases, there are too many "coincidences" and correlations for it to be ignored or discarded. If mercury were the only substance available to combat various health conditions and sicknesses, nobody could fault the dentist or physician, who carefully weighs the potential harm against the possible good before making a decision for its use. Such is not the case. There is no life threatening situation that only mercury can overcome. There is no life threatening situation that requires your dentist to put amalgam fillings in your teeth; there are other suitable materials available.

Why the powers that be persist in their defense of this highly toxic, dangerous substance I will never know. I also cannot understand how we, the patients, have calmly accepted health professionals administering this poison to us, cloaked in the name of "Silver Amalgam", when we know it has the potential of causing irreparable damage to some of us.

As the title to the chapter indicated, there are three questions that we will try to provide some answers to in the following sections.

I.
MERCURY IN MY BODY?

In the previous chapters I have explained in some detail how mercury vapor is released by the dental amalgam. I have also discussed how we inhale this vapor and how we swallow or convert the particles that result from corrosion and abrasion of the amalgam.

Mercury from the dental filling can also travel down through the tooth into our bodies. Once the dentist has cleaned out the decay in the cavity, he prepares it for the filling material by first placing a liner and base into the cavity. This is a resin material that is supposed to seal the cavity and prevent any of the metals in the amalgam filling material from working their way into the pulp and subsequently down through the root into the bone and surrounding tissues.

The protective effectiveness of the seal is quite controversial. Early investigations claimed that they were effective and prevented any passage of the metals into the pulp. However, later studies using radioactive mercury amalgam fillings have shown, by tracing the radioactive mercury, that it does migrate into the pulp. Another study, done by O'Brien and Ryge in 1978, concluded that the sealer will only delay the entry of the mercury into the pulp. The pulp canal extends to the end of the root and has a restricted opening at the very end. This opening permits the body to provide blood and nutrients to the pulp (which is composed of tissue, blood, and nerves) and to the tooth, which in effect keeps the tooth "alive".

If mercury or any of the other metals in the amalgam get into the pulp, they then have a way of getting out of the tooth and into the alveolar bone and the surrounding tissues that support the teeth, where they can then easily migrate to other locations in the body.

Mercury is cytotoxic. This means it acts as a toxin or an antibody and has a specific poisonous effect on the cells. Bleeding gums and alveolar bone loss, which results in loosening of the teeth, are both classic signs of mercury toxicity. Of course these conditions can also be caused by germs or bacteria but according to Till in 1978, who used germ free animals in his experiment, mercury in amounts released from amalgam fillings could produce the same signs plus inflammation of the tissues surrounding a tooth. (This is sometimes called gingivitis, pyorrhea, or periodontitis).

Another very interesting entry route into the body was pointed out by Stock in 1935. He found that some of the mercury vapor coming from the dental amalgams entered the nose. There it was absorbed by the mucosa, and passed rapidly into the brain. It was found in the olfactory lobe and tract (where we have our sense of smell) and in the pituitary gland. A very intriguing study would be to see how many of the millions of people who have some degree of smell impairment also have amalgam fillings? Mats Hanson, a Swedish neurobiology researcher, and others in Sweden, have found that lead, thallium, viruses, and toxins are taken up by the nerve endings and transported to the brain and spinal cord by the "Axon Transport System". (This is a process of a nerve cell by which impulses travel away from the cell body). They are presently investigating their theory that mercury acts in the same manner.

II.
WHERE DOES IT GO?

Once inside the body, where does the mercury go? More importantly, I suppose, would be the question of how mercury moves around in our bodies. It travels by way of biological pathways. In effect, these pathways represent the "road maps" that provide routes for different substances to move along in getting from one point to another.

Scientists have established the fact that mercury has an affinity or attraction for thiols. A thiol is any organic compound containing a univalent radical called a sulfhydrl and identified by the symbol -SH (sulfur-hydrogen). What this really is saying, is that a thiol can attract one atom of mercury in the ionized form and have it combine with itself. It also means, because it is a radical, that it can enter into or go out of this combination without any change.

Amino acids are the building blocks from which the proteins of all organisms are built. The amino acid Cysteine has a sulfhydrl (-SH) as an integral part of its structure and can be found in both the interior and exterior of proteins. Cysteine is always contained in globular proteins and it is this protein that is involved in a tremendous number of functions in the body. Nearly all of our enzymes are made of globular protein and other globular proteins function to transport oxygen, nutrients, and inorganic ions in the blood. Globular proteins also serve as antibodies in our immune system, while others are in hormones or as components of membranes and ribosomes.

When we view the last statement in relation to the fact that cysteine, with its thiol (-SH) component, is a part of all globular proteins and that mercury is attracted to thiols, it is easy to see how mercury can move around in our bodies.

Some of the potential biological pathways for thiols to combine with the mercury ion are:

1. Tissue cell receptor sites. Whenever cysteine is present

on the exterior of a cell membrane, the potential exists for combining.

2. Hormones and Enzymes. All are proteins, so those with a readily accessible thiol group have the capability of combining with the mercury ion.

3. Erythrocytes. These are our red blood cells and they have a hemoglobin content which transports oxygen and iron. Hemoglobin contains 60 times as much thiol as does the human blood plasma. This fact gives it a high potential for combining with the mercury ion. In fact, anemia is frequently encountered in those individuals suffering from mercury intoxication. (anemia represents a reduction in the number of red blood cells contained in 100 milliliters of blood)

4. Glutathione. This is a protein having a specific combination of 3 amino acids, which is called a tripeptide. The important thing here is that one of the amino acids is cysteine with its thiol group and that glutathione is present in high concentrations in all cells. There is quite a bit of research going on at the present time, exploring glutathione and its functions, particularly in its role with selenium and mercury. Both of these metals can bind to the thiol group of glutathione. In fact, both are competing for the same binding sites. The difference being that when selenium combines with glutathione it becomes an essential component of several enzymes in the body, and when mercury binds to glutathione it tends to inhibit or prevent these same enzymes from being formed.

One enzyme in particular that mercury affects is glutathione peroxidase. This enzyme is very important to us because it helps combat or neutralize certain substances (that are normal by-products of metabolism), that, if not controlled would destroy a great number of our cells. When our bodies are deficient in selenium it also means that there is less selenium available to compete with the mercury and, as a result, more mercury ions will bind with the glutathione. This can only serve to aggravate a bad situation.

Another very important discovery was that one of the enzymes necessary to make insulin work in our bodies is made from glutathione. In one form of diabetes, the body has plenty of insulin available, however, it doesn't seem to have any effect on controlling the blood sugar level. Some researchers are currently looking into the possibility that the presence of mercury combined with the enzyme prevents it from doing its normal job of making the insulin active. As you can see, the large amount of glutahathione available in our bodies provides a great thiol pathway for mercury.

5. Coenzyme 'A' and Succinyl Coenzyme 'A'. These are considered by some to be the most important enzymes in the human body and are intimately involved in the way the body converts (metabolizes) glucose (blood sugar) into energy. Because thiol groups are present, we also have the potential pathway for mercury. This, of course, could then have an impact on our energy levels because the mercury has the capability of disrupting or reducing the amount of energy we can produce from glucose.

6. Myosin. Myosin, which contains thiol groups, is the most abundant protein in our muscles. Together, with another protein called Actin, they are responsible for the contraction and relaxation of muscle. The importance of this is that with the thiol group present in our muscles, it then makes it possible for the mercury ion to also be present. The presence of mercury could possibly affect the normal sequence of contraction and relaxation, disturbing the rhythm and causing problems in muscle control. One of the side effects of this action could be tremors, which also happens to be a frequent symptom of mercury intoxication.

7. Cholinergic receptors in heart muscle. As we discussed in an earlier chapter, nerve impulses travel along segments of nerve fibers. To get from one segment of nerve to the next one, the impulse has to get across the synapse, or junction, of the two nerve endings. One group of nerves allows the impulse to "fire" across the junction through the use of a substance derived from choline which is called acetylcholine. Acetylcholine, in effect, becomes a bridge across the junction of the two nerves permitting the impulse to get across. However, every impulse that goes across the junction, uses up the acetylcholine that was in the junction. So before another impulse can get across, some more acetylcholine has to be manufactured and placed back in the junction. This requires a special enzyme which has a thiol group

as a part of it. Therefore, we are once again looking at a potential thiol/mercury pathway; only this time, it is involved with our nerve transmission system.

One way our heart muscles get nerve impulses transmitted to them, so that they can stay regulated, is through the cholinergic receptors (which also contain thiol groups) of the acetylcholine nerve system. So, anything that could inhibit or reduce the effectiveness of the enzyme that makes the acetylcholine, could also possibly affect our heart beat. Scientists know that the mercury ion can combine with the thiol group in the enzyme that makes acetylcholine and reduce the amounts available for insuring continuous uninterrupted transmission of nerve impulses.

Remember also, that the myosin in our heart muscles is responsible for contraction and relaxation dependent upon the nerve impulse received, and that this too, is where the mercury ion can cause a mixup of signals.

All three of these mechanisms, operating together, could possibly be the reason that an irregular heart beat is a frequently seen symptom in mercury toxicity.

8. Factor XIII. This is a protein that is involved in the processes of blood coagulation. As you can imagine, because of its coagulation function in our blood, Factor XIII is available throughout our entire body: outside our red blood cells in the plasma; inside our red blood cells, and also in the placenta. Factor XIII is normally not active and is only activated when there is a need to assist in controlling normal coagulation of the blood, wound healing, placental retention, etc. In its activated form it is designated as Factor XIIIa and in this form it is characterized as a thiol enzyme. This again means we have another potential mercury/thiol pathway.

There is some extremely exciting research being done regarding this compound. One recent paper demonstrated that mercuric ions can react with Factor XIIIa, resulting in inhibition of its activity. Because of this, there have been some theories advanced that it may possibly be involved in tumor growth and metastasis.

9. Thioredoxin. This is another protein in the body that has pairs of thiol (-SH) groups attached, which of course makes it

another potential mercury/thiol pathway. This particular protein is extremely important to us because it is intimately involved in the creation of DNA. DNA (deoxyribonucleic acid) is the carrier of all the genetic information of a cell. Without DNA, the cells could not reproduce exact copies of themselves. Researchers have shown that mercury, when combined with the thiol groups in thioredoxin, can cause an inhibition of the enzyme that results in its inactivation, which they have been unable to reverse.

I hope I haven't confused you by trying to explain in very abbreviated terms some of the most complex biochemical functions performed within our bodies. This is why we all owe such a debt of gratitude to those dedicated researchers who spend years and even lifetimes unraveling all these beautiful mysteries about how the most complicated processes of life really work.

Although we have only explained about the thiol groups, there are other compounds that mercury has an attraction or affinity for. These are chloride ions, amines, and amino acids. All of these in the right situations can combine with the mercury ion and each in their own way affect various body functions and processes.

The important issue for all of us to remember about the potential biological pathways is that they provide highways and routes that permit mercury to travel all over our bodies upsetting very delicate intricate life giving or sustaining functions, in the process. Don't let anyone tell you "there's no way in the world mercury can hurt you in the small doses that may come off your amalgam fillings".

III.
HOW LONG DOES IT STAY?

We have already touched on how it gets in and once it is in, what the different potential biochemical pathways are. Let's explore how it is distributed throughout the body and where it is usually stored or retained.

How, and where, mercury accumulates is a very complex problem that is influenced by many different factors. The degree of absorption is different for the various forms of mercury. For example, mercury vapor is almost completely absorbed into the body, whereas particles of elemental mercury that may be swallowed are poorly absorbed. The role of biotransformation and methylation must also be considered. Your diet, nutritional status, and biochemical individuality are all involved to a degree. For instance, if your diet is rich in foods containing Vitamin C, Cysteine, and Selenium, it is very possible that of the amount of mercury absorbed into the body you would accumulate much less than the person whose diet or body content is low or deficient of these particular nutrients.

Perhaps the most important aspect of where mercury will accumulate depends on the amount of binding material available within an organ or structure. By this I mean, that if the kidney tissues have a great number of thiols present at all times, then they have a built-in capability to accumulate a lot of mercury which has an affinity for thiols.

Consequently, as the mercury moves around the body in our blood and plasma, it will tend to accumulate in those locations that normally have large resident populations of thiols or other substances to which mercury is attracted.

Within the broad category of reactive sulfhydryls, scientists have also found that some have a greater affinity for mercury than others. Dependent upon the form of mercury, especially the forms such as mercury vapor and methylmercury that have the capability of readily passing through membranes, accumulation is going to be determined by the availability and degree of attraction to mercury contained in or at the host location.

Although the foregoing is a vast oversimplification of a tremendously complex problem and researchers are still trying to determine exactly how mercury is distributed to specific locations for which the above rationale does not seem to fully apply, they do know from their research where it accumulates.

The primary or target organs for accumulation of mercury are: kidneys, heart muscle, lungs, liver, brain, and red blood cells. Other storage areas or depots are the thyroid, pituitary, adrenals, spleen, testes, bone marrow, skeletal muscle and intestinal wall.

Some of the differences related to the form of mercury and its ability to accumulate in various locations or compartments are important. Elemental mercury vapor and organic mercury compounds possess the ability to pass through the blood/brain and placental barriers. Because of this ability to penetrate into the brain and placenta, mercury vapor and methylmercury (organic mercury) have the potential of causing the most serious toxic effects.

Mercury vapor also seems to have the ability to penetrate rapidly into all tissues, thereby giving it a fairly uniform distribution pattern. This same capability also results in initial accumulations in the brain that are very high in comparison to the uniform distribution elsewhere. Under normal excretion patterns, mercury vapor will tend to accumulate in the kidneys as it is released from other tissues. However, the brain level remains relatively high, because its release from this particular area has been shown to be very slow. In fact, there have been known cases where mercury retention in the brain has been shown to exist for 10 years or more after the last exposure. In one of those cases, the individual had only been exposed to mercury vapor one time. When he died 13 years after this single exposure, the autopsy revealed relatively high levels of mercury still present in his brain.

Although methylmercury also penetrates the blood/brain barrier its distribution between the brain, kidneys and blood seems to be more uniform. It also tends to have a greater distribution in the red blood cells rather than the plasma whereas mercury vapor will be more uniform in its distribution between red blood cells and plasma. Methylmercury seems to have a particular affinity for distribution and retention in the brain. Like mercury vapor, it too has extremely long retention times in the brain. Sugita in a 1978 paper reported brain retentions of 18–22 years for methylmercury.

A special relationship regarding mercury distribution exists between the mother and the fetus. Much higher levels of methylmercury have been reported in cord blood versus that contained in maternal blood. In animal experiments it has also been shown that there is a much higher accumulation of mercury in the fetal brain tissue than in the maternal brain tissue.

The overall question of retention and excretion is extremely difficult. Like everything else about the toxicity of mercury, scientists are continually discovering and publishing new findings. We could simply say that mercury has a half-life of X number of days, and leave it at that. If we did that, we would be obscuring a very important point.

Utilizing rats in their experiments, Rothstein and Hayes identified three different phases of excretion that have a significant role in retention and cumulative body burden. The first phase is rapid and depletes about 35% of the retained mercury from a single dose in a few days. The second phase is much slower, having a half-life of 30 days, which depletes another 50% of the originally retained dose. The last phase applies to the remaining 15% of the dose and has a half-life of approximately 100 days.

Dr. Clarkson in his 1972 paper expressed the opinion that the last phase would play an extremely important role in determining the total body burden that might be accumulated over time. Concluding that rats having some exposure to mercury on a daily basis would accumulate the metal throughout their life spans, continually adding to their total body burden.

It is apparent from that statement, that we should all be justifiably concerned with the potential for continuous daily exposures to mercury that may be related to our amalgam fillings.

REFERENCES

SECTION I

1. O'Brien, W. J., and Ryge, G., (Editors) An Outline of Dental Materials. W. B. Saunders Co., Philadelphia, 1978.

2. Till, T., Quecksilberabgabe aus Amalgamfullungen und Munddysbakterie als Ursache Parodontaler Abbauerscheinungen. Zahnartzl Welt, Vol 87, page 1076, 1978.

3. Stock, A., Naturwissenschaften, Vol 23, pages 453–456, 1935.

SECTION II

1. Lehninger, A. L., Principles of Biochemistry. Worth Publishers Inc., 1982.

2. Cooke, R. D., et al. Calcium and Thio Reactivity of Human Factor XIII. Biochemical Journal, Vol 141, Issue 3, pages 675–682, 1974.

3. Sarausa, M. M., et al. Human Factor XIII—Metal Ion Interactions. Journal of Biologic Chemistry, Vol 257, Issue 23, pages 14102–14108, 1982.

SECTION III

1. Sugita, M., The Biological Half-Time of Heavy Metals. The Existence of A Third and Slowest Component. International Archives of Occupational Health, Vol 41, page 25, 1978.

2. Rothstein, A., and Hayes, A. D., Journal of Pharmacology and Experimental Therapy, Vol 130, pages 166–176, 1960.

3. Clarkson, T. W., (See No. 3 Argument 2, Chapter 4).

CHAPTER 7

PATHOLOGY
DOES MERCURY CAUSE ANY CHANGES IN
OUR TISSUES AND ORGANS?

The other chapters all lead to this one on Pathology. That is because it wouldn't matter how mercury got into the body, or where it went, or how long it stayed, if it didn't do any damage to our tissues and organs. Pathology is the branch of medicine that is concerned with any structural or functional changes in tissues and organs of the body that are caused by disease, or might in themselves cause a disease.

We keep calling mercury a toxic poison. It's now time to provide a definition of those two words. Dorland's Illustrated Medical Dictionary defines poison as "any substance which, when ingested, inhaled or absorbed, or when applied to, injected into or developed within the body, in relatively small amounts, by its chemical action may cause damage to structure or disturbance of function". Toxic is defined as "pertaining to, due to, or of the nature of a poison". When mercury is classified as toxic or a poison, it is pretty serious business because it means it has the potential to damage our tissues and organs and disturb their normal functions.

The subject is extremely complex, as I am sure you can easily imagine. So much so, that thousands of books and articles have been published on individual facets of each aspect of this branch of medicine. However, in relation to the total amount of information available on pathology, mercury comprises only a minor amount. Accordingly, this chapter can only hope to focus on some of the key pathological findings on mercury contained in the published literature. Please understand that I am not attempting to convey the idea that everything presented pertains to mercury amalgam fillings. However, it would be a disservice to anyone reading this book to NOT include critical information indicating the potential damage to the human body that mercury can cause, regardless of the source.

Notwithstanding all the latest scientific equipment and laboratory techniques, there is more that is not known about mercury's effects on the body, than is known. Each day, scientists and researchers all over the world are adding to the store of knowledge on the pathology of mercury and it's possible involvement in so many known diseases of unknown origin. That is why unraveling the mysteries of "Heavy Metal Toxicities" could be the greatest medical breakthrough since the beginning of time.

Each of the major areas of concern is outlined in the subsequent sections of this chapter.

I.
CENTRAL NERVOUS SYSTEM (CNS)/BRAIN

The central nervous system consists of the brain and spinal cord nervous systems.

The blood-brain barrier is described as an obstruction or a membrane (thin layer of tissue) which acts to separate the blood from the essential functional elements of the central nervous system. Its purpose is to regulate or filter the exchange of metabolic material between the brain and the blood. (Steinwell, 1961; Steinwell and Klatzo, 1966; Dorland's Medical Dictionary)

Without this barrier to filter the substances that otherwise might get in, the brain would be totally vulnerable to the thousands of man-made chemicals that we are routinely exposed to in our food, drink, and environment, and to those toxins produced within our own bodies.

Researchers have shown that mercury will penetrate the blood-brain barrier and enter the nerve cells from the blood. (Berlin and Ulberg, 1963; Ware, Chang and Burkholder, 1974).

These discoveries establish the potential for neurotoxic effects (poisonous or destructive to nerve tissue). With that as a background, let's look at some of the pertinent findings:

1. The blood-brain barrier is more than just a physical barrier. It also has a regulatory function by controlling the passage of selected biological substances from the blood to the nervous system. (Broman and Steinwall, 1967).

2. When less than one part per million (<1.0 ppm) of mercury ions are absorbed into the blood stream they can impair the blood-brain system within hours, permitting subsequent entry of substances contained in the plasma that would normally be barred or excluded. (Chang and Hartman, 1972; Ware, Chang and Burkholder, 1974).

3. Yoshino et al, in 1966 studied the biochemical changes in rat nervous systems resulting from mercury intoxication and concluded that poisoning by alkylmercury compounds might be the reason that he observed a selective inhibition of protein. Several other researchers doing independent studies confirmed Yoshino's observations that after mercury intoxication there is a great reduction of amino acids being incorporated into brain tissue. (Steinwall, 1969; Steinwall and Snyder, 1969; Cavanagh and Chen, 1971). The significance of this action was hypothesized to be an impairment of the blood-brain barrier.

4. All mercury compounds cause the same type of structural damage to the brain, but to different extents. (Chang, 1977; Schaumberger and Spencer, 1979; Gallagher and Lee, 1980).

5. Methylmercury produces rather complex changes in the metabolic responses of the brain, suggesting that the coordination of energy metabolism to functional activity (metabolic control) had been impaired. The alterations in intermediary metabolism in the brain occur at doses of methylmercury far below those producing overt toxicity in rats. (Bull and Lutkenhoff, 1975).

6. Human autopsy studies have revealed brain damage in persons who had been exposed to organic and inorganic mercury compounds. (Hay et al, 1963; Chang, 1980).

7. Neurological disturbances consisting mainly of mild tremor, ataxia (failure of muscular coordination and irregular movement), and sensory and visual loss were very prevelant in

the clinical observations of methylmercury poisoning. (Katsuki et al, 1957; Okinaka, 1964; Brown et al, 1967).

8. Gerstner and Huff in 1977 concluded that the symptoms of methylmercury poisoning are a reflection of damage to both the central nervous system and the peripheral nervous system. Rabenstein in 1978 stated that there was a latent period between exposure and the development of symptoms.

9. For long term exposure to mercury vapor, the organ that first exhibits functional disturbance appears to be the central nervous system. The toxic effects are produced after the body converts or transforms the elemental mercury vapor into mercuric ions. (Clarkson, 1968; Rothstein, 1971).

10. Progressive constriction of the visual fields, often progressing to blindness, has been reported repeatedly in almost all significant exposures of humans to methylmercury. (Hunter et al, 1940; Garman et al, 1975; Bakir et al, 1980).

11. Impaired hearing to complete deafness was detected in more than 33% of the affected adults and 50% of the affected children during the 1971 Iraqi epidemic of methylmercury poisoning. (Amin-Zaki et al, 1978).

12. Komulain and Tuomisto in 1981, utilizing rats for their experiments, found that methylmercury, even at low concentrations, inhibited the uptake in synaptic nerve endings in the brain of the neurotransmitters dopamine, noradrenaline, and serotonin. (A neurotransmitter is a compound secreted by a conducting cell of the nerve from its terminal which is bound by the next conducting cell and in this manner is carried along, transmitting a nerve impulse. Dopamine is a hormone like neutrotransmitter compound that is required as an intermediate step in the chemical process the body goes through to make noradrenaline. Noradrenaline is also called norepinephrine and is a hormone secreted by the conducting cell of the nerve that also acts as a neurotransmitter compound to the peripheral nerves and to some parts of the central nervous system. Serotonin is another nerve substance that acts to constrict blood vessels in many parts of the body including the central nervous system). In essence what the researchers are saying is that methlymercury prevented these neurohormones/transmitters from getting into

the central nervous system in the brain and performing their normal functions.

13. This last report appears to have a correlation to the information provided in 12 above. Parkinson's Disease is a degenerative disease of the central nervous system characterized by tremor, rigidity, hypokinesia (abnormally decreased mobility), ataxia (failure of muscle coordination), dysarthria (speech control impairment), and mental depression. The disease seems to be related to a depletion or impairment in the use of dopamine by those central nervous system neurons that require dopamine for activation. Ohlson and Hogstedt in 1981 studied six cases that had been diagnosed as having Parkinson's Disease and who had all been determined to have had exposure to mercury. The authors recommended further exploration of a possible association between exposure to mercury and Parkinson's Disease.

The studies related above and in the subsequent sections of this chapter, should only serve to reinforce the insidious nature of mercury and its ability to cause serious health problems. It can produce symptomatology that makes it extremely difficult, if not impossible for the clinician to clearly identify "it" as the primary causative factor.

We readily admit that live studies of the human brain and central nervous system present researchers with insurmountable problems. However, the ability to gain epidemiological data does not. There is an urgent and desperate need for investigative studies that separate and classify patients into two distinct categories; those with mercury amalgam fillings and those without. Studies of this type could help many people worldwide who are afflicted with health problems for which medical institutions can find no identifiable cause. Certainly it is not an unreasonable request to have these same institutions explore the mercury amalgam relationship through the simple collection of statistics on the living and those who die while under their care.

II.
RENAL FUNCTION

Renal and nephric are other medical terms used to identify the kidneys. These are the two organs in the body that have the function of filtering the blood. The kidneys are designed to filter out and excrete in the form of urine, the end-products of body metabolism. The kidneys also perform the important function of regulating the concentrations of hydrogen, sodium, potassium, phosphate and other ions in the extracellular body fluids (not inside the cell). These extracellular fluids include blood plasma, lymph, and cerebrospinal fluids.

There seems to be general agreement among researchers that mercury, which is also filtered and excreted by the kidneys, has the potential of causing serious injury to these vital organs:

1. Nephrotoxicity from mercury exposure is well documented in scientific literature: Friberg, 1959; Rodin and Crawson, 1962; Joselow, et al, 1967; Selye, 1970, and Wisniewska, et al, 1970; just to mention a few. (Nephrotoxic is defined as being destructive to kidney cells).

2. Pathological biochemical damage was found in the kidneys of various animals who had been exposed to mercury in concentrations below those levels presently considered as relatively safe for humans by the World Health Organization. Another significant fact was that the animals appeared outwardly healthy. (Nicholson et al, 1983).

3. Chronic exposure to mercury vapor may cause proteinuria (an excess of serum proteins in the urine, also called albuminuria) which may progress to a nephrotic syndrome. (Friberg et al, 1953; Kazantzis et al, 1962; Joselow and Goldwater, 1967). Dorland's Illustrated Medical Dictionary defines nephrotic syndrome as "a condition characterized by massive edema, heavy proteinura, hypoalbuminemia, and peculiar susceptibility to intercurrent infections". Intercurrent is defined as "breaking into and modifying the course of an already existing disease".

4. Kidney damage may result from excessive exposure to mercury as manifested by the nephrotic syndrome of edema, proteinuria, and the presence of cells in the urine. Such damage

may or may not be accompanied by an elevated mercury level in the urine. The nephrotic syndrome may be the only manifestation of mercury intoxication. In more severe cases of kidney damage, renal failure and oliguria may develop, leading to complete anuria. (Occupational Exposure to Inorganic Mercury, OSHA, 1973). (Oliguria is a condition where you are not excreting enough urine in relation to the amount of fluids you drink. Anuria is the condition where you are not excreting any urine).

III.
CARDIOVASCULAR

A recently published study by Abraham et al, 1984, demonstrated that mercury amalgam fillings can contribute to a higher level of mercury in the blood. It was felt that these increases resulted from inhaled mercury vapor reaching the blood via lung absorption. Two previous studies on this same subject failed to show any positive connection between amalgams and blood mercury levels. However, as in all studies dealing with human test subjects, results can be affected by a great many factors. In the study conducted by Abraham and his co-workers, they attempted to take a great many of these factors into consideration, which could be why their results were positive. Their results also correlated very well with another study done in 1982 by Kuntz et. al. that involved pregnant women and the measurement of maternal and cord blood mercury levels deemed attributable to amalgam fillings. (This study is discussed in greater detail in a subsequent section).

The real tragedy of this is not that mercury amalgam increases mercury blood levels, but rather that the true health hazards of this phenomenon have not been fully explored and documented by medical science. The potential of mercury to have a bearing on the genesis of our major health problems has been known for centuries yet its potential for subtle and insidious damage has never been fully examined and documented by medical science.

This is a round about way of saying that although some research has been done on the possible relationship of mercury to cardiovascular disease, it must be considered as extremely small in relation to the billions of dollars that have been expended and are continuing to be spent searching for reasons and cures for this No. 1 Killer. 3½ Billion Dollars was spent in 1981 on Heart By-Pass Surgery alone, which has nothing to do with finding the underlying cause that created the problem in the first place.

Some of the studies that have been done are reported here:

1. Mercury adversely affects the functioning of the heart. (Joselow, et al, 1972; Mantyla and Wright, 1976: Trakhtenberg, 1968).

2. Mercuric chloride blocked the vascular response to injections of norepinepherine and potassium chloride in rat mesenteric vascular beds (the large blood supply contained in the membranes attaching the small intestines to the back wall of the body). The mechanism of this action was related to a direct effect of mercury on blocking the entry of calcium ions into the cytoplasm (a site inside the cell where most of the chemical activities take place). (Oka, et al, 1979). Norepinpherine is normally released when the body detects low blood pressure. The nerves in the arterial muscles get the message and respond by contracting the muscle, increasing the blood pressure. Potassium and calcium are both involved in the process of muscular contraction.

3. Exposure to mercury compounds has been found to induce cardiovascular impairment. (Chang, 1977; Gerstner and Huff, 1977)

4. Myocardial infarction (this involves the death of cells and their coagulation in the muscular tissues of the heart, usually caused by a deficiency of blood due to a restriction in the flow of coronary arterial blood), coronary artery thromboarteritis (this is a collection of blood factors consisting of platelets and fibrin that bind with other cellular elements, some of which could be metal ions, to form a thrombus, which is similar to a clot, causing an obstruction to blood flow), coronary artery aneurysm (a weakening of the cell wall letting it push out forming a sac), AV Block (causing an interruption of the proper sequence of contraction of the chambers of the heart. The block means restricting the entrance of blood into the chambers), and premature ventricular contractions (early contraction of the lower heart

chamber) have been found in mucocutaneous lymph node syndrome (MLNS) patients. (Orlowski and Mercer, 1980; Adler et. al., 1982).

Some researchers of MLNS or Kawasaki Syndrome (Dr. Kawasaki first identified the syndrome) are attempting to find a relationship between mercury and the disease. Kawasaki was unable to confirm the presence of mercury in his patients and Orlowski and Mercer could not identify a source of mercury in their patients but did discover significant urinary excretion levels of mercury in six of their patients. It may surprise many of the readers to learn that this is not a syndrome that only affects people living in foreign countries. From 1971 to 1980, the Center For Disease Control (CDC) has received information about more than 400 cases of MLNS occurring in the United States. In a report in the Feb 25, 1983 issue of the Morbidity and Mortality Weekly Report, the CDC reported that since October 1982 there had been four outbreaks of Kawasaki Syndrome (MLNS) consisting of 43 cases in 4 states over a 3-month period. The CDC position is that there is no known cause for this syndrome. Coronary artery aneurysms are present in 17% to 31% of all the cases and the case-fatality ratio is 1%.

It is entirely possible that the signs and symptoms associated with this syndrome could be attributable to something other than mercury. However, based on the very limited amount of research accomplished that attempts to correlate mercury exposure to MLNS or KS, I am at a loss to understand how the hypothesis that mercury may be involved can be ignored without further exploration.

5. Electocardiographs (ECG's) were studied from 42 victims of organic mercurial poisoning. The ECG's were abnormal in all 42 cases. (Dahan and Orfaly, 1964).

6. A 1983 article by Carmignani, Finelli and Boscolo, reported a study utilizing mercury-exposed rats. They demonstrated that chronic exposure to inorganic mercury affects cardiovascular function by interfering with the blood pressure reflexes and/or the reactivity of catecholamines. (Catecholamines are adrenaline, also called epinephrine, dopamine, and norepinephrine, which are hormone like compounds that function as neurotransmitters). The effects of norepinephrine on

the alpha-adrenergic receptors of the cardiovascular system were significantly reduced. (Alpha-adrenergic receptors are thought to be located in the nerve fibers of the sympathetic nervous system. In this instance we are referring to their location in heart and arterial muscles where they have a direct effect on the amount of norepinephrine released in response to signals of low blood pressure. Norepinephrine would normally cause a contractile response in the arterial muscle to increase pressure.)

7. Clinical and experimental reports suggest that prolonged exposure to mercuric chloride increases sympathetic activity (Cheek, et al, 1959) and potentiates vascular response to epinephrine (Axelrod and Tomschick, 1958).

Epinephrine or adrenaline, as most of us know it, stimulates the sympathetic nervous system. It increases blood pressure, stimulates the heart muscle accelerating the heart rate and increases the blood output of the heart. Carmigani, et al, 1983, also investigated this potentiating vascular response of epinephrine that had been reported earlier. They suggested that the presence of the mercury ion reduces the amount of calcium available within the arterial muscle. Calcium is required for the contractile response of the arterial muscle and because there was a reduced amount available when the mercury ion was present, this would then cause the artery to open or dilate more than usual, resulting in a drop in blood pressure instead of the normal response to epinephrine which is an increase in blood pressure. Their conclusions also support the mercury/calcium findings of Oka, et al, reported in 2 above.

IV.
THE ENDOCRINE SYSTEM

The critical importance of the endocrine system warrants that we have some description of the overall system before we start discussing mercury's relationship to it.

Endocrine means to secrete inward or internally. Exocrine means just the opposite, to secrete outwardly through a duct. The endocrine system is composed of glands and other structures that have the capability to produce substances (hormones) and secrete or release them directly into the blood or lymph circulatory systems (lymph, derived from tissue fluids, is gathered from all parts of the body and returned to the blood through its own circulatory system). Once released into the blood, hormones have a specific effect on another organ or part of the body.

The organs or glands that have this endocrine capability are the pituitary, adrenals, thyroid and parathyroid, pancreas, gonads, the pineal body and the paraganglia (a collection of cells that can store and release the neurotransmitters epinephrine and norepinephrine).

The endocrine glands control or influence almost all body processes through the secretion of their hormones. The glands are under the direct or indirect control of the nervous system. When the receptors in the glands, or storage sites, receive appropriate signals from the nerves, the glands secrete their chemical substances in the blood which then function upon reaching their target organs or structures to maintain or restore metabolic balance. Hormones exert specific effects in the body on metabolism, growth, maturation, development and organ function. Hormones are generally produced as required, are inactivated as they are utilized, and are then excreted in the urine.

There are essentially three classes of hormones: steroid, peptide (protein), and amino acid. The steroid and peptide hormones have short half-lives varying from 5 minutes to 100 minutes, and circulate in the plasma. The short half-life usually means that the hormones have to exert their biological effects fairly rapidly. Factors controlling this are the availability of a receptor and an interaction between the hormone and the receptor. The other significant controlling factor is the amount or the circulating level of the hormone.

The steroid hormones are generally lipid soluble and bind to globulin proteins in the plasma for transport. The protein or polypeptide hormones are generally water soluble and circulate unbound in the plasma. The amino acid hormones have characteristics in-between the steroid and peptide and some have half-lives of up to a week. They can also attach to multiple binding proteins for transport in the plasma.

Anything that is introduced into the body that increases, or decreases, or affects the biological activity of these hormones can in turn cause the delicate balance control mechanisms of the body to go astray. The body cannot react properly which results in these imbalances causing such conditions as infantilism (too little growth hormone secreted), gigantism (too much growth hormone secreted), diabetes (too little insulin hormone secreted), to Hyperthyroidism (too much thyroxin hormone secreted). The extremes of some of these imbalances can be death unless, as in the case of diabetes, a synthetic hormone is available.

Now, let's look at some of the research findings in regard to the relationships of mercury to our endocrine glands and hormones:

1. The pituitary and thyroid glands in humans display an affinity for the accumulation of mercury. (Suzuki, et al, 1966; Kosta, et al, 1975).

2. The concentrations of mercury in the pituitary and thyroid glands were much higher than that found in the kidney, brain, or liver tissues in humans. (Kosta, et al, 1975).

3. Goldman and Blackburn in their 1978 article, describe experiments utilizing rats that were given mercuric chloride and radioactive iodine, the purpose being to determine whether the mercury affected the thyroid gland's ability to uptake iodine. (Iodine is an essential nutrient the thyroid utilizes in the production and secretion of its hormones). Rats given oral doses of mercuric chloride over a 90 day period displayed signs of mercury poisoning together with a reduction in uptake of the radioactive iodine. There was also a decrease in the secretion rate of thyroid hormones. After 90 additional days during which the rats had no exposure to mercury, the depression of thyroid function did not improve and was concluded to be permanent and irreversible.

Trakhtenberg (1974), in his experiments using radioactive iodine, showed there were significant increases in the uptake of the radioactive iodine by the thyroid even under low quantities of mercury. "Persons who show increased uptake of the isotope, as a rule, show symptoms of thyroid gland enlargement, finger tremors, emotional sensitivity, etc." As one of his conclusions Trakhtenberg states, "low mercury concentrations produce hormonal shifts and thyroid dysfunction.'' This was also found to be true with the pituitary and adrenal glands.

5. Animals poisoned with methylmercury exhibit stress intolerance and decreased sexual activity, suggesting both adrenal and testicular dysfunction. The data indicated impairment of the adrenal and testicular steroid hormone secretions. The authors concluded that the tissue levels of methylmercury required to cause the observed endocrine abnormalities of the adrenals and testes might be somewhat lower than those associated with overt neurological dysfunction. (Burton and Meikle, 1980)

6. Burton's study, outlined above, confirmed previous findings of Khera in 1973 and Stoewsand, et al, in 1971, that methylmercury diminished sexual activity in birds and mammals.

7. Methylmercury intoxication causes subnormal fertility and spermatogenesis (the process of formation of the sperm) in rats. (Lee and Dixon, 1975; Thaxton and Parkhurst, 1973)

8. Methylmercury intoxication causes impaired growth in rats. Diamond and Sleight, 1972; Kojima and Fujita, 1973)

9. Alomar et al, in 1983 related a case involving a 52 year old farmer who was diagnosed as having contact dermatitis and Addison's disease, attributable to mercury in the soap he was using. Addison's disease is due to reduced function of the adrenal glands and is usually fatal. Some of the symptoms are progressive anemia, low blood pressure, diarrhea and digestive disturbances.

It is evident from the limited information available that mercury has the potential of upsetting our delicate hormonal balance, either through increasing/decreasing the quantities secreted or decreasing the biological activity of the hormone itself.

If, in our wildest imagination, there exists the remote possibility that mercury, induced into our bodies from dental amalgam has the potential to affect our endocrine system, then some positive action is required. It is imperative that persons, institutions, and governmental agencies, who are involved in the decision making that dictate the continued use of mercury amalgam for dental restorations provide adequate scientific proof to support any claim that amalgam is harmless. As a minimum, the following actions should be taken:

1. Adequate priorities and funding must be provided for medical scientists to fully explore and reach a documented decision that either refutes or supports the claim of amalgam's harmlessness.

2. The opposition to finding the truth must be stilled. We can no longer accept 150 years of continued use as "prima facie evidence" that amalgam is harmless. As a part of this effort, a public apology should be issued to those dentists who made their decision to stop using amalgam based on available scientific evidence. These individuals have been placed in professional jeopardy by those opposed to finding the scientifically correct answer.

To those of you who have such a dentist, count your blessings. You have a dedicated health care provider who is more interested in your personal health and well being than he is in the orthodoxy of the establishment or the peer pressure that ensues.

V.
THE IMMUNE SYSTEM

Immunology is perhaps the most complicated of all the biomedical sciences. It becomes more complicated each year as researchers discover more about the immune system and its interdependence with so many other systems, organs, and functions of the body which previously had been thought to be unrelated.

The development of sophisticated laboratory equipment and techniques has permitted researchers to explore and learn more about our immune system. More knowledge has been gained in the last 20 years than everything that had been previously learned since the beginning of time. One important fact that is emerging from all of this newer research is that the immune system may be involved in the pathogenesis of all diseases.

For you to be able to understand the nature of the possible relationships that mercury has to our immune system, it is necessary that you have a general idea of how the system works.

There is a general principle underlying the living organism's ability to survive which is called homeostasis. It can be described as a state of stability, or remaining always the same, or being in balance. We endure from conception to death because of this principle.

For every action that takes place within our bodies, there is a balancing action that takes place to maintain homeostasis. For example, cells that make up our skin are constantly dying, but for every cell that dies, the body makes a new one to replace it. Every time your heart muscle contracts to push blood out into your arteries and veins, there is an opposite action that makes the same muscle relax to permit more blood to enter the chamber.

The immune system works in the same manner. For every foreign bacteria or germ cell that gets into our body, we are supposed to have a defense cell available to neutralize or destroy it. For every stimulus that is given for a defender cell to destroy an invader, there must be a counter stimulus to stop sending more defender cells. For every foreign invader that is destroyed, there must be some way to remove it from the body. For every one of the defense cells that is used up in the fight, a new one must be produced to be available for the next battle.

For every action there has to be an interaction and counter action. All of this is accomplished by a communications network that is so sophisticated and complex that science has only been able to unravel part of it.

What are the components of our complicated immune system and how do they function in the never-ending battle to protect or defend us? There are two major body environments in which the system must be able to operate. In the first is on the inside and on the outside surface of the cell. This is called Cellular Immunity. The second is in the fluids of our body, such as the blood, lymph, saliva, tears, and in the secretions of the mucous membranes in our nose, vaginal tract, and small intestine. This is called humoral (fluid) immunity.

Most of us are familiar with the two major classifications of cells (red blood cells and white blood cells) found in blood. Within the white blood cell classification (also called leukocytes) we have one type of cell that is the central cell in our immunity system. These are called lymphocytes.

There are two types of lymphocytes designated as T lymphocytes or B lymphocytes. These are usually referred to simply as T cells and B cells. T cells get their name from the fact that they are either produced in the Thymus Gland or their development is influenced by the Thymus Gland. B cells are named after bone marrow because it is thought to be the site where they are produced.

Both T cells and B cells have specific functions to perform in our immune system.

T cells are responsible for a great number of the functions involved in cellular immunity. To do this they are endowed with special qualities that permit them to migrate or travel to the site of infection or problem and once there to be able to independently move through tissue and capillary walls. They also function to defend against certain microorganisms such as disease producing bacteria that may get inside cells, fungi, poxviruses like small pox, and are supposed to provide antitumor immunity.

B cells, and their offspring the plasma cells, are responsible for humoral immunity. To accomplish this, the B cells produce certain proteins that circulate in the plasma. These are called antibodies or immunoglobulins. The immunoglobulins are the protein molecules that are possessed of the antibody capability. It is this antibody capability that makes the system so unique. Regardless of the number of different foreign microorganisms, the system can produce an antibody specifically tailored to attack every one of them.

The foreign substances that get into the body are called antigens. They are so named because they cause the system to produce an antibody so precise that it can only recognize one particular antigen. This is an amazing and extraordinary capability that the immune system possesses. There are literally millions of different antigens that your body may be exposed to, yet the immune system has the capability of producing a specific antibody for each antigen. Although we won't elaborate on it, there are 5 classes of immunoglobulins. Each class is identified by a letter suffix that relates to its specific biological properties and capabilities: IgA, IgD, IgE, IgG and IgM.

Let's look at an example of how it all works together.

Each germ has its own antigen. When one of them gets into the body, the body has the capability to differentiate between its own cells and a foreign cell. So, when the body senses the intruder, it starts the sequence of actions in motion that will neutralize or destroy the invader. The T cell recognizes the germ, or carrier of the antigen, and sends a stimulating message to the B cell, which then recognizes the antigen fraction of the germ. The B cell then tells the immunoglobulin to produce the specific antibody for the antigen. The B cell, with its antibody and with help from a special class of T cell (called a helper cell), surrounds, or engulfs, the antigen and neutralizes or destroys it and in the process also kills the germ. Once the job is completed, another type of T cell (called a suppressor cell) gets a stimulating message and proceeds to suppress further production, and eliminate most of the unused antibody. Some of the antibody remains alive, and in the blood, so that if the specific antigen ever returns there will be a built in immunity to it. The used up B cells, with immunoglobulin and dead germs, are then passed along to the liver and kidneys where they are excreted in the urine and feces.

The same sequence of events usually takes place when we have an allergic reaction. Except that in the case of allergic reactions, the type of B cell immunoglobulin antibody that normally responds is IgE, which has the capability to cause the body's cells at the site of invasion or contact to release histamine. Histamines are what cause the red, or flushed, skin reaction that is evoked when an allergic person is exposed to an allergen. This is why antihistamine drugs are sometimes effective in controlling allergic reactions. Allergen is another term used to describe any antigen that stimulates IgE production.

Now that background information on the immune system has been provided, I will list some of the reported relationships between mercury and leukocytes and the immune response.

1. High frequencies of chromosomal aberrations were observed in cultured lymphocytes from humans that had been exposed to mercury. (Vershaeve, et al, 1976; Popescu, et al, 1979; Skerfving, et al, 1970, 1974).

A chromosome is that portion of the cell containing a thread of DNA which contains many genes and functions to store and transmit genetic information. It is in this manner that lymphocytes are able to reproduce clones or exact duplicates of themselves. Aberration means that there is an alteration of the genetic information when it is transferred; it could mean the duplication, loss, exchange or alteration in the sequence of the genetic material which ordinarily would be reproduced as an exact duplicate of the original sequence. Any aberration of the chromosome constitutes a biological change that is thought to be one of the earliest actions leading to decreased immunity and increased susceptibility to disease.

2. The toxic effects of methyl and ethyl mercury on white blood cells included chromosomal breakage, alteration of mitosis (replication of chromosomes), and death of cells. (Fiskesjo, 1970)

3. Lymphocytes from mercury-diseased rats showed a significant decrease in their ability to stimulate chromosomal replication compared with lymphocytes from control animals (no exposure to mercury).

Mercury-induced anti-nuclear antibodies (specific to the nucleus or core of leukocyte cells in the blood and tissues) were found in more than 90% of the experimental animals.

Thymus and spleen lymphocytes from mercury diseased animals produced a migration inhibitory factor reducing the ability of the lymphocytes to travel to other locations in the body. This was determined by incubating the lymphocytes with the two antigens utilized in the test. Lymphocytes from control animals, not exposed to mercury, did not produce the migration inhibition factor.

A relative loss of suppressor T-cell function was found in rats with mercury-induced immune complex glomerulopathy. (a disease of that section of the kidneys called the glomeruli which is composed of blood vessels). Administration of low doses of inorganic mercury over a prolonged period induces an immune complex glomerulopathy in experimental animals. (Weening et al, 1980).

4. Mercury suppresses the primary humoral (antibody) immune response. (Blakley, et al, 1980; Koller, 1973, 1975 and Koller, et al, 1980).

5. Experiments were performed in the laboratory utilizing lymphocytes from individuals who showed no prior evidence of allergy to mercury, and lymphocytes from individuals who had known allergies to mercury. When mercuric chloride was added

to both cultures of lymphocytes, there was a transformation of the blast cells (immature cells) in both groups. The organic mercurial compound Merbromin (you know it as mercurochrome) also caused blast cell transformation, but Thimerosal (merthiolate) did not, even though it was determined to be cytotoxic (having the effect of a toxin or antibody that has a specific toxic action upon cells of special organs) (Schopf, et al, 1967; Caron, et al, 1970).

6. In a recent article published in the May issue of the Journal of Prosthetic Dentistry, Dr. David W. Eggleston, describes experiments involving three patients that demonstrated the ability of dental amalgam and dental nickel alloys to adversely affect the quantity of T-lymphocytes. In his experiments, Dr. Eggleston measured the T-lymphocyte percent of total lymphocytes in the patients' blood before and after the insertion and removal of dental amalgam and nickel-base alloys. In the first patient removal of six amalgam fillings resulted in a 55.3% increase in the number of T-lymphocytes. Reinsertion of four amalgam restorations resulted in a decrease in the T-lymphocyte count of 24.7%. Similar changes were obtained on the other two patients. Dr. Eggleston concludes by stating "Further research may determine the frequency and magnitude of T-lymphocyte reduction and alteration by dental materials."

There are a great number of other papers demonstrating the impact that mercury can have on our immune response and potential allergic reactions. The studies cited above adequately make the point that mercury can be a potent antigen and allergen as well as possessing the capability to alter our body's basic defense mechanisms to infection and disease. The implications of Dr. Eggleston's work provides additional urgency to reclassify the population into those with metal fillings, those without fillings and those with non-metal fillings. All future medical studies must consider this fact when attempting to determine the cause of disease in the human body.

VI.
ORAL CAVITY

The oral cavity could be utilized to make a great TV commercial advertising the outstanding health benefits available from the use of mercury. This of course is said with tongue in-cheek and bleeding gums. If you don't believe me just look at some of the benefits listed in the literature:

1. Mercury poisoning may be acute or chronic, but the systemic (affecting the body as a whole) reactions in the acute form are so serious that the oral features need not be considered. Chronic mercurialism (mercury poisoning) occurs after prolonged contact with mercurial compounds in a variety of situations, including therapeutic use of these compounds and as an occupational hazard.

The oral cavity suffers seriously in mercurialism and evidences numerous characteristic signs and symptoms (but they are not necessarily ones that can always be used to make a diagnosis of mercurialism). There is an increased flow of saliva and a metallic taste in the mouth. The salivary glands may be swollen, and the tongue is sometimes enlarged and painful. Hyperemia (excess of blood) and swelling of the gingiva (gums) are occasionally seen. The oral mucosa (mucous membranes) is prone to ulcerations on the gingiva, palate (the roof of the mouth) and tongue. In severe cases, pigmentation of the gingiva may occur. Loosening of the teeth, even leading to exfoliation (falling out), has been reported.

A toxic reaction from absorption of mercury in dental amalgam has been reported on a number of occasions. Frykholm (1957), after a thorough review of the literature and numerous studies on the absorption and excretion of mercury, concluded that the amount of estimated exposure to mercury from dental amalgam is not sufficient to cause mercury poisoning in the conventional sense. Nevertheless, this exposure may suffice to bring about allergic manifestations in patients sensitive to mercury. (Shafer et al, 1974, A Textbook of Oral Pathology) I bet you didn't think they taught about mercury in dental school.

2. Poisoning from the inhalation of mercury vapors is characterized by metallic taste, stomatitis (inflammation of the oral

mucosa), foul breath, gingivitis (inflammation of the gum tissue), and excessive salivation. Necrosis (death of the tissue) of the alveolar processes (the bony sockets in which the roots of the teeth are attached), loosening of the teeth, and discoloration of the gingival margins may appear later. (Goodman and Gillman's, The Pharmacological Basis of Therapeutics, 1980)

3. Two cases of Multiple Polypous Hyperplasias (growths, polyps, protruding from the mucous membrane that result from an abnormal increase of normal cells in normal arrangement in the tissue) of the oral mucosa that disappeared after removal of the amalgam fillings. Both patients had diseased lymph nodes in the neck. Metal ions were found in the biopsied tissues. (Bergenholtz, 1965)

4. Local inflammatory reactions induced by amalgam fillings have been observed in the gingival tissue. (Zander, 1957; App, 1961; Freden, et al, 1974).

5. Mercury levels of over 1200 micrograms per gram of tissue were found at the root tips of teeth having both gold and amalgam restorations. Up to a few hundred micrograms per gram of tissue were found at the root tips of those teeth having only amalgam restorations. The levels recorded increased with time and did not come from food. (Till and Maly, 1978).

I apologize for my opening remarks in this section. It certainly isn't a joking matter.

The information cited above, provides substantiation that the mercury can migrate out of the amalgam, as well as evidence of its potential toxicity. The point of departure between the believers and non-believers is the statement by Frykholm "the estimated exposure to mercury from dental amalgam is not sufficient to cause mercury poisoning in the conventional sense". This same philosophy is essentially embraced by the ADA and responsible government agencies. The fallacy of the philosophy is that it cannot be substantiated by scientific proof because sufficient research on the pathology and biochemistry of micro doses of mercury (micromercurialism) has not been done. In fact, there is not even a definition of the word micromercurialism contained in the medical dictionaries that I checked. In their minds, the condition doesn't even exist.

VII.
MERCURY TOXICITY IN THE HUMAN REPRODUCTIVE CYCLE
MOTHER? EMBRYO? FETUS? INFANT?

There appears to be an ever increasing number of children born who are either mentally or physically impaired, or both. Medical science is conducting some investigations into the phenomenon in relation to some of the more prevalent diseases that are manifested in the newborn. However, it is certainly an area of exploration worthy of a major national effort.

From the time of fertilization until birth, the offspring is dependent upon the mother for all sources of nutrition, as well as for routes of elimination for metabolic wastes. There are essentially four major areas that are considered to be critical or determining, in the outcome of fetal development: 1. The mother's nutritional status; 2. The structural and functional quality of the placenta; 3. The genetic makeup of the offspring; and 4. The presence of physical, chemical, or mechanical insults to mother and child during pregnancy. (McClintic, 1975).

It was previously thought that the placental membrane (it used to be called placental barrier) protected the fetus from possible damage from any of the potentially toxic drugs or substances that might be present in the mother's blood. Medical scientists now know that this was a myth. This is probably why the name was changed from barrier to membrane. The widely publicized Thalidomide disaster in 1961 demonstrated clearly that the passage of toxic substances from mother to fetus did occur and that the results could indeed be manifested in deformities that were tragic.

We are talking of very delicate mechanisms in the development of the embryo (first 2 to 8 weeks) and fetus (subsequent to 8 weeks). Medical scientists are learning more each day about the potential pathological and neurological changes that may occur in fetal development as a direct result of maternal nutritional deficiences and/or the introduction into the fetal blood of micro levels of drugs and foreign chemical substances previously thought to be harmless. Some examples of this are: Mental retardation in the offspring resulting from a maternal deficiency of iodine during the first two months of pregnancy (please recall Professor Trakhtenberg's findings regarding thyroid uptake of iodine in the presence of mercury); anticonvulsant drugs given to epileptic mothers may result in an increased incidence of cleft lip and palate, cardiac abnormalities, chromosomal aberrations, and mental deficiencies; and the maternal use of barbiturates may result in the development of hyperexcitability of brain neurons.

There is another area of concern dealing with the potential dangers associated with the drug and foreign chemicals contained in mother's milk. This area is coming under increased scientific scrutiny because, here again, there is apparently only a very limited filtering mechanism at work to preclude the introduction of these drugs and chemicals during suckling of the infant. The list of substances that may be passed to the child in this manner is truly amazing. Dr. Arena, in his 1979 book on poisons, cited approximately 150 different drugs and chemical substances excreted in human milk, covering everything from alcohol and caffeine to mercury.

The potential toxicity to the mother and her offspring associated with her total body burden of mercury cannot be ignored. Obstetricians are now cautioned to advise their patients to avoid all exposure to mercury. The scientific studies that follow clearly demonstrate the wisdom of that advice. Please pay particular attention to the study by Dr. Kuntz and his colleagues that, for the first time, clearly implicates dental fillings as contributing to the mother's total body burden of mercury:

1. Morphological (forms and structure), behavioral, and physiological (normal functioning) studies show methylmercury as having an injurious effect on the fetal nervous system even at levels which are considered not to be toxic in adults. (Reuhl and Chang, 1979; Clarkson et al, 1981; and Marsh, et al, 1980).

2. The concentration of methyl mercury in fetal blood is about 20% higher than in the mother. (Tejning, 1968).

3. The following is an abstract of the paper published by Dr. Kuntz and his co-workers in 1982. I personally consider it to be a landmark study worthy of the closest scrutiny by all health care providers, regardless of specialty. "Fifty-seven prenatal patients with no known exposure to the element mercury, or any of

its compounds, were observed for change in whole blood total mercury concentration from the initial prenatal clinic examination through delivery and postpartum hospitalization. On hospital admission for labor and delivery, whole blood total mercury averaged 1.15 parts per billion, compared to 0.79 parts per billion from the first prenatal clinic visit; these levels represent a 46% increase and significant difference in maternal concentration of a substance previously recognized for its peculiar ease at crossing the placental barrier. Previous stillbirths, as well as history of birth defects, exhibited significant positive correlation with background mercury levels. Search of the literature of the last 5 years revealed no other report of cohort heavy metal surveillance throughout pregnancy. (Kuntz, W. D.; Pitkin, R. M.; Bostrom, A. W.; and Hughes, M. S. Published in the American Journal of Obstetrics and Gynecology, Vol 143, issue 4, pages 440–443. 1982).

Dr. Kuntz concluded their study with the following statement: "Among obstetric-related historical factors, a significant association was found between previous stillbirths and mercury levels in both maternal and cord blood. Previous malformed infants significantly correlated with prenatal background mercury levels. Except for smoking early in pregnancy, none of the historical data reflecting possible mercury exposure correlated significantly with blood levels, although patients with large numbers of dental fillings exhibited a tendency to higher maternal blood mercury levels."

What is urgently needed now is for the major medical agencies and institutions to confirm and expand these findings presented by Dr. Kuntz and his associates. It also reinforces a point I made earlier regarding the necessity of considering the presence or non-presence of dental amalgam fillings if findings and conclusions derived from medical and scientific studies of humans are to be considered accurate and credible.

4. Symptoms of congenital Minamata (methylmercury) Disease included intelligence disturbances, primitive reflexes, disturbances of body growth, speech difficulties, limb deformity, hyperkinesia (hyperactivity resulting from brain damage or psychoses) and pyramidal symptoms (skilled movements, especially those of speech and those involving the hands and fingers). Mi-

crocephaly (abnormally small head/mental retardation) was present in approximately 60% of cases. The outcome was deformed, mentally retarded children and a mortality rate of approximately 7%. (Tedeschi, 1982)

5. Thirty-two infants prenatally (prior to birth) exposed to methylmercury and their mothers were studied and evaluated over a 5 year period after the Iraqi methylmercury epidemic. Although the mothers' symptoms usually improved, the damage to the fetal and infant nervous system appeared to be permanent: 1. The infants exhibited clinical manifestations of various degrees of damage to their central nervous system. 2. Ten of the 32 infants had cerebral palsy. 3. Nine of the 32 died within three years. This mortality rate of 28% compared to a 6% mortality rate in the control group (no prenatal exposure to mercury). 4. Twelve of the surviving 23 had delayed mental development; 18 showed delayed speech development; 16 showed delayed motor development; 6 had an abnormally small head circumference; and 21 exhibited hyperreflexia (exaggeration of reflexes). (Amin-Zaki and Clarkson, et al, 1979).

There are dozens of other studies that I could cite, but they all essentially confirm the findings reflected in the studies I have used. They all confirm the potential hazards of mercury exposure during pregnancy. The medical profession recognizes this fact also. Obstetricians are cautioned to advise their patients to avoid all exposure to mercury. In light of the implication of dental amalgam as a source of mercury, it would seem reasonable to also expect the medical profession to advise couples contemplating having a child about this aspect of exposure. Dental amalgam fillings should not be placed or replaced after conception because of the possibility of temporarily increasing the total body burden of mercury.

VIII.
FANTASY LAND
OR REAL PSYCHIATRIC AND BEHAVIORAL MANIFESTATIONS?

It is apparent from the body of literature already mentioned in this book that the brain, with its component central nervous and endocrine systems, has a serious problem coping with the fact that mercury "likes" it so well.

It's like the story about the distant relative who, though uninvited, stops by to "free load" for a week-end and likes it so much that he decides to hang around until someone throws him out. Unfortunately, you only have an efficiency apartment and no matter how much you protest, your relative moves in and makes himself at home.

No matter how hard you try to ignore him and follow your normal way of life, this unwanted visitor is always under foot, getting in your way, and disrupting your regular routine. In fact, you even find him wearing your things and disguising himself to look like you. You get so frustrated you don't know what to do. What's even worse, he now looks so much like you that even some of your long time associates who look to you for advice and guidance, can't tell you apart. They even invite him into their homes to visit. However, they soon become as confused as you, because they can't figure out why you're acting so different. They can't understand why you keep playing practical jokes and tricking them into doing things they never did before.

After feeling frustrated, you become depressed. Nobody seems to understand or even want to believe in you anymore because you are so erratic. In final desperation, you decide you have to seek outside help, and go to your longtime doctor friend and tell him all you need is somebody to help you throw this unwanted visitor out, because you seem powerless to do it by yourself. He can't help, but he has a colleague that might be able to. He sets up a consultation for you with his colleague the psychiatrist, and you pour out your tale, but as intelligent and learned as he is, he doesn't seem to believe you. But, don't blame yourself, it's really his fault because nobody ever told him that the possibility even remotely existed that "unwanted visitors" could ever do this to you or anyone else.

IS THE STORY FACT OR FANTASY? Let's look at some of the facts and you judge for yourself:

1. Symptoms of methylmercury poisoning in man include psychic and behavioral disturbances. (Snyder, 1972; Kojima and Fujita, 1973; Gerstner and Huff, 1977).

2. Sixty-three persons poisoned during the 1971 Iraqi epi-

demic of methylmercury poisoning were examined. Some of the findings were: Headache occurred in 53% of the cases; 51% had sleep disturbances; 45% experienced dizziness; 42% were irritable; 12% suffered from emotional instability; and 6% were diagnosed as having mania and depression. (Damuji et al, 1976).

3. Behavioral abnormalities may occur at mercury levels below those causing clearly identifiable morphological (forms and structures) alterations and may be among the most sensitive indicators of methylmercury induced neurotoxicity (exerting a destructive or poisonous effect upon nerve tissue). (Hughes et al, 1976; Spyker, et al, 1972).

4. In another evaluation study of patients hospitalized during the second epidemic of methylmercury poisoning in Iraq that occurred in early 1972, there appeared to be a significant number suffering from depression. Of the 43 patients in the study, thirty-two (74.4%) were consistently depressed. Clinically depressive symptoms were mild to moderate in degree, consisting mainly of a feeling of depression, lack of interest, deficient concentration, and a wish to be left alone. Mercury binding compounds did not seem to have a significant effect in enhancing recovery from the depressive state. (Maghazaji, 1974).

5. Nine medical laboratory technicians who had been exposed to mercury vapor and dust were investigated. Some of the women were complaining of symptoms which were thought to be neurotic by their physicians until an investigation of three cardiac laboratories revealed significant levels of mercury in the atmosphere. The most common symptoms displayed by the technicians were: irritability, shyness, fatigue, headaches, nightmares, anxiety, tension, depression and forgetfulness. (Ross and Sholiton, 1983).

6. Metallic mercury demonstrates the importance of quantitative measures of motor function in assessing subclinical impairment (lack of positive identifiable symptoms) as well as the lack of sound psychophysiological (having bodily symptoms of an emotional origin) data about the total syndrome of mercury poisoning. Now that exposures in dental offices and laboratories are coming under increased scrutiny, psychologists might be asked what measures of psychophysiological function might help detect subclinical toxicity. Such measures could help to

identify some sources of the psychological complaints accompanying mercury intoxication. We do not have tests to recognize effects on the nervous system. There are virtually no useful tests for preclinical stages and diseases of specific organ systems such as the central nervous system. (Weiss, 1983).

Acceptance of the hypothesis that mercury in micro doses may be involved in the manifestation of psychoses is extremely difficult for the physicians who specialize in this area of medicine. It is too controversial and contrary to the accepted doctrines upon which most diagnoses are based, unless of course there has been an obvious and identifiable source of exposure to mercury. The analogy might be compared to Einstein's theory of relativity. When first expressed, it was beyond the comprehension of most other prominent physicists who maintained it wouldn't work and couldn't be proved. History, of course, proved how right Einstein was. That's where we are with micromercurialism and the art of psychiatry. All that is needed now is the "openmindedness and events" to prove or disprove the hypothesis.

REFERENCES

SECTION I

1. Steinwell, O., Transport Mechanisms in Certain Blood-Brain Barrier Phenomena—A Hypothesis. Acta Psychiatr Neurol Scand, Supplement 150, Vol 36, pages 314–318, 1961.

2. Steinwell O., and Klatzo, I., Selective Vulnerability of The Blood-Brain Barrier in Chemically Induced Lesions. Journal of Neuropathology and Experimental Neurology, Vol 25, pages 542–559, 1966.

3. Berlin, M., and Ullberg, S., Accumulation and Retentions of Mercury in The Mouse. 1. An Autoradiographic Study After A Single Intravenous Injection of Mercuric Chloride. Archives of Environmental Health (Chicago), Vol 6, pages 589–601, May 1963.

4. Broman T., and Steinwall O., Blood-Brain Barrier In: Pathology of the Nervous System. (J. Minckler Editor), Vol 1, Chapter 33. Blakeston. New York, 1967.

5. Chang L. W., and Hartman H. A., Blood-Brain Barrier Dysfunction in Experimental Mercury Intoxication. Acta Neuropathology, Vol 21, pages 179–184, 1972.

6. Ware R. A., Chang L. W., and Burkholder P. M., An Ultrastructural Study on the Blood-Brain Barrier Dysfunction Following Mercury Intoxication. Acta Neuropathology (Berlin), Vol 30, pages 211–224, 1974.

7. Yoshino Y., Mozai T., and Nakao K., Journal of Neurochemistry, Vol 13, pages 1223–1230, 1966.

8. Steinwall O., Brain Uptake of Se75-Selenomethionine After Damage to Blood-Brain Barrier by Mercuric Ions. Acta Neurologica Scandinavica, Vol 45, pages 362–368, 1969.

9. Steinwall O., and Snyder H., Brain Uptake of C^{14}—Cyclo-Leucine After Damage To Blood-Brain Barrier by Mercuric Ions. Acta Neurologica Scandinavica, Vol 45, pages 369–375, 1969.

10. Cavanagh J. B., and Chen F.C.K., Amino Acid Incorporation in Protein During the "Silent Phase" Before Organ-Mercury and P-Bromophenylacetylurea Neuropathy in the Rat. Acta Neuropathology (Berlin), Vol 19, pages 216–224, 1971.

11. Chang, L. W., Neurotoxic Effects of Mercury—A Review. Environmental Research, Vol 14, pages 329–373, 1977.

12. Schaumberger H. H., and Spencer P.S., Clinical and Experimental Studies of Distal Axonopathy—A Frequent Form of Brain and Nerve Damage Produced by Environmental Chemical Hazards. Annals of the New York Academy of Science, Vol 329, pages 14–29, 1979.

13. Gallagher P. J., and Lee R. L., The Role of Biotransformation in Organic Mercury Neurotoxicity. Toxicology, Vol 15, pages 129–134, 1980.

14. Bull R. J., and Lutkenhoff S. D., Changes in Metabolic Reponses of Brain Tissue to Stimulation, In Vitro, Produced By In Vivo Administration of Methylmercury. Neuropharmacology, Vol 14, pages 351–359, 1975.

15. Hay W. J., Richards A. G., McMenemey W. H., and Cumings J. N., Organic Mercurial Encephalopathy. Journal of Neurology and Neurosurgical Psychiatry, Vol 26, pages 199–202, June 1963.

16. Chang L. W., Mercury In: Experimental and Clinical Neurotoxicology. Williams and Wilkins, Baltimore, 1980.

17. Katsuki, et al., On the Disease of Central Nervous System in Minamata District With Unknown Etology With Special References To Clinical Observations. Kumamoto Igakki Zasshi (Suppl 23), Vol 31, pages 110–121, 1957.

18. Okinaka S., et al., Encephalomyalopathy Due To An Organic Mercury Compound. Neurology, Vol 4, pages 68–76, 1964.

19. Brown, et al., Medical Service Journal of Canada, Vol 23, page 1089, 1967.

20. Gerstner H. B., and Huff J. E., Clinical Toxicology of Mercury. Journal of Toxicology and Environmental Health, Vol 2, Issue 3, pages 491–526, 1977.

21. Rabenstein D. L., The Chemistry of Methylmercury Toxicology. Journal of Chemical Education, Vol 55, Issue 5, pages 292–296, 1978.

22. Clarkson, T. W., Biochemical Aspects of Mercury Poisoning. Journal of Occupational Medicine, Vol 10, pages 351–355, July 1968.

23. Rothstein A., Mercaptans, The Biological Targets for Mercurials In: Mercury, Mercurials and Mercaptans. Miller M. W., and Clarkson T. W. Editors, Charles C. Thomas, Springfield, Illinois, 1971.

24. Hunter, et al., Poisoning by Methylmercury Compounds. Quarterly Journal of Medicine, Vol 33, pages 193–206, 1940.

25. Garman R. H., Weiss B., and Evans H. L., Alkylmercurial Encephalopathy in The Monkey (Saimiri Scieureus and Macaca Arctoides) A Histopathologic and Autoradiographic Study. Acta Neuropathology (Berlin), Vol 32, Issue1, pages 61–74, 1975.

26. Bakir, et al., Clinical and Epidemiological Aspects of Methylmercury Poisoning. Postgraduate Medical Journal, Vol 56, pages 1–10, 1980.

27. Amin-Zaki, et al., Methylmercury Poisoning in Iraqi Children. Clinical Observations over 2 Years. British Medical Journal, Vol 1, Page 613, 1978.

28. Komulainen H., and Tuomisto J., Effect of Heavy Metals On Dopamine, Noradrenaline And Serotonin Uptake and Release In Rat Brain Synaptosomes. Acta Pharmacology and Toxicology, Vol 48, pages 199–204, 1981.

29. Ohlson C.-G., and Hogstedt C., Parkinsons Disease and Occupational Exposure to Organic Solvents, Agricultural Chemicals and Mercury—A Case Referent Study. Scandinavian Journal of Work Environment Health, Vol 7, Issue 4, pages 252–256, 1981.

SECTION II

1. Friberg L., Studies on The Metabolism of Mercuric Chloride and Methylmercury Dicyandiamide. Archives of Industrial Health, Vol 20, page 42, 1959.

2. Rodin A. E., And Crawson C. N., Mercury Nephrotoxicity in Rats: I Factors Influencing Localization of Tubular lesions. American Journal of Pathology, Vol 41, pages 297–313, 1962.

3. Joselow M. M., Goldwater L. T., and Weinberg S. B., Absorption and Excretion of Mercury in Man. Mercury Content of "Normal" Human Tissues. Archives of Environmental Health, Vol 15, Page 64, 1967.

4. Selye H., Mercury Poisoning: Prevention by Spironolcatone. Science, Vol 169, pages 775–776, 1970.

5. Wisniewska, et al., Binding of Mercury in Rat Kidney by Metallothionein. Toxicology and Applied Pharmacology, Vol 16, pages 754–763, 1970.

6. Nicholson J. K., et al., Cadmium and Mercury Nephrotoxicity. Nature, Vol 304, pages 633–635, 1983.

7. Friberg, et al., Kidney Injury After Chronic Exposure to Inorganic Mercury. Archives of Industrial Hygiene and Occupational Medicine, Vol 8, pages 149–153, 1953.

8. Kazantzis G., et al., Albuminuria And The Nephrotic Syndrome Fol-

lowing Exposure to Mercury And Its Compounds. Quarterly Journal of Medicine, Vol 31, pages 403–418, 1962.

9. OSHA Job Health Hazard Series: Mercury. OSHA 2234, August 1975.

SECTION III

1. Abraham J. E., Svare C. W., and Frank C. W., The Effect of Dental Amalgam Restorations on Blood Mercury Levels. Journal of Dental Research, Vol 63, Issue 1, pages 71–73, January 1984.

2. Kuntz W. D., et al., Maternal and Cord Blood Background Mercury Levels: A Longitudinal Surveillance. American Journal of Obstetrics and Gynecology, Vol 143, Issue 4, pages 440–443, 1982.

3. Joselow M. M., et al., Mercurialism: Environmental and Occupational Aspects. Annals of Internal Medicine, Vol 76, pages 119–130, 1972.

4. Mantyla D. G., and Wright O. D., Mercury Toxicity in The Dental Office: A Neglected Problem. Journal American Dental Association, Vol 92, pages 1189–1194, 1976.

5. Trakhtenberg I. M., et al. In: Problems of Geohygiene. Baku, page 47, 1968. Cited in Trakhtenberg Chronic Effect of Mercury on Organisms. USDHEW, PHS, NIH, DHEW Publication No. (NIH) 74–473, USGPO Washington D.C., 1974.

6. Oka M., et al., Effect of Mercuric Chloride on The Rat Mesenteric Vascular Bed: Relevance to The Mechanism of Mercury Toxicity. Toxicology and Applied Pharmacology, Vol 51, pages 427–438, 1979.

7. Chang L. W., Neurotoxic Effects of Mercury—A Review. Environmental Research, Vol 14, pages 329–373, 1977.

8. Gerstner H. B., and Huff J. E., Clinical Toxicology of Mercury. Journal of Toxicology and Environmental Health, Vol 2, Issue 3, pages 491–526, 1977.

9. Orlowski J. P., and Mercer R. D., Urine Mercury Levels in Kawasaki Disease. Pediatrics, Vol 66, Issue 4, pages 633–636, 1980.

10. Adler R., et al., Metallic Mercury Vapor Poisoning Simulating Mucocutaneous Lymph Node Syndrome. Journal of Pediatrics, Vol 101, Issue 6, pages 967–968, 1982.

11. Gregg M.B., (Editor). Kawasaki Syndrome—United States. Morbidity and Mortality Weekly Report, Vol 32, Issue 7, pages 98–100, 1983.

12. Gregg M. B., (Editor). Kawasaki Disease—New York. Morbidity and Mortality Weekly Report, Vol 29, pages 61–63, 1980.

13. Dahhan S. S., and Orfaly H., Electrocardiographic Changes in Mercury Poisoning. American Journal of Cardiology, Vol 14, pages 178–183, 1964.

14. Carmignani M., et al., Mechanisms in Cardiovascular Regulation Following Chronic Exposure of Male Rats to Inorganic Mercury. Toxicology and Applied Pharmacology, Vol 69, Issue 3, pages 442–450, 1983.

15. Cheek D. B., et al., The Effect of Mercurous Chloride (Calomel) and

Epinephrine (Sympathetic Stimulation) on Rats. The Importance of the Findings to Mechanisms in Infantile Acrodynia. Pediatrics, Vol 23, page 302, 1959.

16. Axelrod J., and Tomschick R., Enzymatic O-Methylation of Epinephrine and Other Catechols. Journal of Biological Chemistry, Vol 233, pages 702–705, 1958.

SECTION IV

1. Williams R. H., (Editor). Textbook of Endocrinology, 6th Edition, 1981. W. B. Saunders Co., Philadelphia.

2. Suzuki T., et al., Affinity of Mercury to the Thyroid. Industrial Health, Vol 4, pages 69–75, 1966.

3. Kosta L., et al., Correlation Between Selenium and Mercury in Man Following Exposure to Inorganic Mercury. Nature (London), Vol 254, pages 238–239, 1975.

4. Goldman M., and Blackburn P., The Effect of Mercuric Chloride on Thyroid Function in the Rat. Toxicology and Applied Pharmacology, Vol 48, pages 49–55, 1979.

5. Trahktenberg I. M., (See No. 5, Section III)

6. Burton B. V., and Meikle A. W., Acute and Chronic Methyl Mercury Poisoning Impairs Rat Adrenal and Testicular Function. Journal of Toxicology and Environmental Health, Vol 6, pages 597–606, 1980.

7. Khera K. S., Reproductive Capability of Male Rats and Mice Treated With Methyl Mercury. Toxicology and Applied Pharmacology, Vol 24, pages 166–177, 1973.

8. Stoewsand, et al., Eggshell Thinning in Japanese Quail Fed Mercuric Chloride. Science, Vol 173, pages 1030–1031, 1971.

9. Lee I. P., and Dixon R. L., Effects of Mercury on Spermatogenesis Studied by Velocity Sedimentation Cell Separation and Serial Mating. Journal of Pharmacology and Experimental Therapeutics, Vol 194, pages 171–181, 1975.

10. Thaxton J. P., and Parkhurst C. P., Abnormal Mating Behavior and Reproductive Dysfunction Caused by Mercury in Japanese Quail. Proceedings Society of Experimental Biology and Medicine, Vol 144, pages 252–255, 1973.

11. Diamond S. S., and Sleight S. D., Acute and Sub-Chronic Methylmercury Toxicosis in the Rat. Toxicology and Applied Pharmacology, Vol 23, pages 197–207, 1972.

12. Kojima K., and Fujita M., Summary of Recent Studies in Japan on Methylmercury Poisoning. Toxicology, Vol 1, pages 43–62, 1973.

13. Alomar A., et al., Addison's Disease and Contact Dermatitis from Mercury in Soap. Contact Dermatitis, Vol 9, Issue 1, page 76, 1983.

SECTION V

1. Stites D. P., Stobo J. D., Fundenberg H. H., and Wells J. V., Basic and Clinical Immunology, 4th Edition, 1982. Lange Medical Publications, Los Altos, CA.

2. Williams R. H., (See No. 1, Section IV)

3. McClintic J. R., Physiology of The Human Body. John Wiley & Sons, Inc., N.Y., 1975.

4. Homberger F., Hayes J. A., and Pelikan E. W., (Editors). A Guide to General Toxicology. Karger AG, Basel, Switzerland, 1983.

5. Verschaeve L., et al., Genetic Damage Induced by Occupational Low Mercury Exposure. Environmental Research, Vol 12, pages 306–316, 1976.

6. Popescu H. I., et al., Chromosome Aberration Induced by Occupational Exposure to Mercury. Archives of Environmental Health, Vol 34, Issue 6, pages 461–463, 1979.

7. Skerfving S., Hansson K., and Linstren J., Chromosome Breakage in Humans Exposed to Methylmercury Through Fish Consumption. Archives of Environmental Health, Vol 21, pages 133–139, 1970.

8. Skerving S., et al., Methylmercury-Induced Chromosome Damage in Man. Environmental Research, Vol 7, pages 83–98, 1974.

9. Fiskesjo G., The Effect of Two Organic Mercury Compounds on Human Leukocytes In Vitro. Hereditas, Vol 64, pages 142–146, 1970.

10. Weening J. J., Chapter 4, Mercury Induced Immune Complex Glomerulopathy: An Experimental Study. Van Dan Denergen, 1980.

11. Blakley, et al., The Effect of Methylmercury, Tetraethyl Lead and Sodium Arsenite on The Humoral Response in Mice. Toxicology and Applied Pharmacology, Vol 52, pages 245–254, 1980.

12. Koller L. D., Immunosuppression Produced by Lead, Cadmium and Mercury. American Journal of Veterinary Research, Vol 34, page 1457, 1973.

13. Koller L. D., Immunotoxicology of Heavy Metals. International Journal of Immunopharmacology, Vol 2, pages w69–279, 1980.

14. Schopf E., Schultz K. H., and Gromm M., Transfcrmationen Und Mitosen Vun Lymphozyten In Vitro Durch Quecksilber (11)-Chlorid. Naturwissenschaften, Vol 54, page 568, 1967.

16. Caron G. A., Poutala S., and Provost T. T., Lymphocyte Transformation Induced by Inorganic and Organic Mercury. International Archives of Allergy and Applied Immunology, Vol 37, pages 76–87, 1970.

SECTION VI

1. Frykholm K. O., On Mercury From Dental Amalgam Its Toxic and Allergic Effects and Some Comments on Occupational Hygiene. Acta Odontologica Scandinavica, Vol 15, Supplement 22, pages 1–108, 1957.

2. Schafer, et al., A Textbook of Oral Pathology. W. B. Saunders Co., Philadelphia, 1974.

3. Goodman and Gillman's, The Pharmacological Basis of Therapeutics. 6th Edition, 1980. Macmillan Publishing Co., Inc. New York.

4. Bergenholtz A., Multiple Polypous Hyperplasias of the Oral Mucosa With Regression After Removal of Amalgam Fillings. Acta Odontologica Scandinavica, Vol 23, Issue 2, pages 111–131, April 1965.

5. Zander, H. A., Effect of Silicate Cement and Amalgam on the Gingiva. Journal American Dental Association, Vol 55, page 11, 1957.

6. App G. R., Effect of Silicate, Amalgam and Cast Gold on the Gingiva. Journal of Prosthetic Dentistry, Vol 11, page 522, 1961.

7. Freden H., et al., Mercury Content in Gingival Tissues Adjacent to Amalgam Fillings. Odontologica Review, Vol 25, Issue 2, pages 207–210, 1974.

8. Till T., and Maly K., Zum Nachweis Der Lyse Von Hg Aus Silber-Amalgam Von Zahnfullungen. Der Praktesche Arzt, Vol 32, page 1042, 1978.

SECTION VII

1. McClintic J. R., (See No. 3, Sect V)

2. Arena, J., Poisoning, 4th Edition, 1979. Charles C. Thomas, Springfield, Illinois.

3. Kuntz N. D., et al., Maternal and Cord Blood Background Mercury Levels: A Longitudinal Surveillance. American Journal of Obstetrics and Gynecology, Vol 143, pages 440–443, 1982.

4. Reuhl K. R., and Chang L. W., Neurotoxicology, Vol 1, pages 21–55, 1979.

5. Clarkson T. W., et al., Dose-Response Relationships for Adult Prenatal Exposures to Methylmercury. In: Measurement of Risks, G. G., and Mialle H. D., (Editors). Plenum, New York, 1981.

6. Marsh D. O., et al., Fetal Methylmercury Poisoning: Clinical and Toxicological Data on 29 Cases. Annals of Neurology, Vol 7, pages 348–453, 1980.

7. Tejning S., Mercury Levels in Blood Corpuscles and in Plasma in "Normal" Mothers and Their New-Born Children, Report 68 02 Z from Dept of Occupational Medicine, University Hospital, Lund Sweden, Lung Stencils, 1968.

8. Tedeschi L. G., The Minamata Disease. American Journal of Forensic Medicine and Pathology, Vol. 3, Issue 4, pages 335–338, 1982.

9. Amin Zaki L., et al. and Clarkson T. W., et al., Prenatal Methylmercury Poisoning. American Journal Disabled Children, Vol. 133, pages 172–177, 1979.

SECTION VIII

1. Snyder, R. D., The Involuntary Movements of Chronic Mercury Poisoning. Archives of Neurology, Vol 26, pages 379–381, 1972.

2. Kojima, K., and Fujita, M., Summary of Recent Studies in Japan on Methylmercury Poisoning. Toxicology, Vol. 1, Issue 1, pages 43–62, 1973.

3. Gerstner H. B., and Huff, J. E., Clinical Toxicology of Mercury. Journal of Toxicology and Environmental Health, Vol. 2, Issue 3, pages 491–526, 1977.

4. Damuji S. F., and The Clinical Committee on Mercury Poisoning, Intoxication Due to Alkyl-Mercury Treated Seed—1971–1972-Outbreak in Iraq Clinical Aspects, Bulletin World Health Organization, Vol. 53, (Suppl), page 65, 1976.

5. Spyker, J. M., et al., Subtle Consequences of Methyl Mercury Exposure: Behavioral Deviations in Offspring of Treated Mothers. Science, Vol. 177, pages 621–623, 1972.

6. Maghazaji, H. I., Psychiatric Aspects of Methylmercury Poisoning. Journal of Neurology, Neurosurgery and Psychiatry, Vol. 37, Issue 8, pages 954–958, 1974.

7. Ross, W. D., and Sholiton, M. C., Specificity of Psychiatric Manifestations in Relation to Neurotoxic Chemicals. Acta Psychiatry Scandinavia, Vol. 67, Suppl 303, pages 100–104, 1983.

8. Weiss, B., Behavioral Toxicology and Environmental Health Science. Opportunity and Challenge for Psychology. American Psychologist, Nov 1983, pages 1174–1187.

CHAPTER 8

MICROMERCURIALISM
AND SIGNS AND SYMPTOMS
MERCURY CAN PRODUCE

Although there are references to micro doses and micromercurialsm in several places in the book, I haven't attempted to define it previously. Micromercurialism was first described by Professor Stock in 1926 on the basis of psychological changes observed in persons chronically exposed to low concentrations of atmospheric mercury. Professor Trakhtenberg in his 1969 monograph called the micromercurialism defined by Stock an "asthenic-vegetative syndrome".

Dorland's Illustrated Medical Dictionary does not list micromercurialism or carry the asthenic-vegetative syndrome under their listing of established syndromes. However, it does define the terms: asthenic is defined as "pertaining to or characterized by asthenia." Asthenia is defined as "lack or loss of strength and energy; weakness." Of the six major categories of asthenia defined, the three considered most pertinent to our discussion are: "asthenia gravis hypophyseogenea, a pituitary dysfunction marked by emaciation, anorexia, constipation, amenorrhea, hypothermia, hypotonia, and hypoglycemia. Myalgic asthenia, a condition in which the general symptoms are a sensation of general fatigue and muscular pains. Neurocirculatory asthenia, a symptom complex characterized by the occurrence of breathlessness, giddiness, a sense of fatigue, pain in the chest in the region of the precordium, and palpitation. It occurs chiefly in soldiers in active war service, though it is seen in civilians also. Called also effort syndrome, cardiac neurosis, DaCosta's disease or syndrome, anxiety neurosis, neurasthenia, cardiasthenia, cardiac neurasthenia and cardioneurosis." Vegetative is defined as "functioning involuntarily or unconsciously, as the vegetative nervous system; (an old term for the autonomic nervous system)."

Professor Trakhtenberg states in his monograph that Professor Stock characterized micromercurialism symptoms in three groups according to their degree of intensity of the phenomenon. "First degree micromercurialism results in lowered work capacity, increased fatigue, light nervous excitability. Often in the second degree there is swelling of the nasal membranes, progressive weakening of memory, feelings of fear and loss of self-confidence, irritability, headaches. Simultaneously there may be catarrhal symptoms and upper respiratory discomfort, changes in the mucous membranes of the mouth, bleeding gums. Sometimes there are feelings of coronary insufficiency, shivering, quickening pulse, and a tendency toward diarrhea. Third degree micromercurialism is characterized by symptoms approaching those of regular mercurialism, but to a lesser degree. The basic symptoms of this stage are: headaches, general weakness, sleeplessness, decline in intellectual capacity, depression. Among other signs are tears, diarrhea, frequent urination, a feeling of pressure in the cardiac region and shivering." Please keep in mind that Professor Stock stated his findings in 1926.

Professor Trakhtenberg also cited reports by A. M. Gel'fand (1928), and A. N. L'vov (1939) that focus on the difficulty of diagnosing micromercurialism. Gel'fand found that sometimes mercury poisoning in patients was mistaken for other diseases and L'vov cited cases of micromercurialism misdiagnosed as neurasthenia, hysteria, etc. He further noted that although there were only a few cases of chronic mercury poisoning reported among mercury industry workers, qualified pathologists frequently reported the phenomenon of micromercurialism among this same class of mercury workers.

Professor Trakhtenberg concludes in his monograph that clinical micromercurialism shows characteristic symptoms of its own in addition to the classical symptoms of chronic mercury poisoning. These were attributed to disturbances in the cortical centers of the central nervous system and are manifested by functional changes in organs of the cardiovascular, urogenital, or endocrine systems. (NIOSH, Occupational Exposure to Inorganic Mercury, 1973).

Again, and as most scientists that have studied micromercurialism have concluded, further study, toxicological experimentation and additional clinical observations are needed.

SIGNS AND SYMPTOMS
ELEMENTAL MERCURY VAPOR EXPOSURE

1. **Psychological disturbances (erethism):**
   Irritability
   Nervousness
   Shyness or timidity
   Loss of memory
   Lack of attention
   Loss of self-confidence
   Decline of intellect
   Lack of self control
   Fits of anger
   Depression
   Anxiety
   Drowsiness
   Insomnia

2. **Oral Cavity Disorders:**
   Bleeding gums
   Alveolar bone loss
   Loosening of teeth
   Excessive salivation
   Foul breath
   Metallic taste
   Leukoplakia
   Stomatitis
   Ulceration of gingiva, palate, tongue
   Burning sensation in mouth or throat
   Tissue pigmentation

3. **Gastrointestinal Effects:**
    Abdominal cramps
    Gastrointestinal problems, colitis
    Diarrhea
4. **Systemic Effects:**
    Cardiovascular:
    Irregular heartbeat (tachycardia, bradycardia)
    Feeble and irregular pulse
    Alterations in blood pressure
    Pain or pressure in chest
    Neurologic:
    Chronic or frequent headaches
    Dizziness
    Ringing or noises in ears
    Fine tremors: hands, feet, lips, eyelids, tongue
    Respiratory:
    Persistent cough
    Emphysema
    Shallow and irregular respiration
    Immunological:
    Allergies
    Asthma
    Rhinitis
    Sinusitis
    Lymphadenopathy, especially cervical
    Endocrine:
    Subnormal temperature
    Cold, clammy skin, especially hands and feet
    Excessive perspiration
    Muscle weakness
    Fatigue
    Anemia
    Hypoxia
    Edema
    Loss of appetite (anorexia)
    Loss of weight
    Joint pains

5. **Severe Cases:**
>   Hallucinations
>   Manic-depression

ORGANIC MERCURY EXPOSURE

1. **Earliest Symptoms**
>   Fatigue
>   Headache
>   Forgetfulness
>   Inability to concentrate
>   Apathy
>   Depression
>   Outbursts of anger
>   Decline of intellect

2. **Later Findings:**
>   Numbness and tingling of hands, feet, lips
>   Muscle weakness progressing to paralysis
>   Dim or restricted vision
>   Hearing difficulty
>   Speech disorders
>   Loss of memory
>   Incoordination
>   Emotional instability
>   Dermatitis
>   Renal damage
>   General central nervous system dysfunctions

3. **Late Symptoms**
>   Coma
>   Death

The problem with a listing of signs and symptoms is that they can apply to so many other diseases, syndromes, or impaired health conditions. I caution everyone not to jump to conclusions. However, I also urge anyone with a mouth full of silver amalgam fillings and a collection of the signs and symptoms listed, who has repeatedly sought medical help in determining the cause, and has not received a conclusive diagnosis or treatment, to pursue the matter further.

It won't be easy. The prevailing attitude within the medical and dental communities will probably subject you to a "professorial" lecture on the ridiculousness of a question like "Doctor could the mercury in my amalgam fillings have any bearing on my condition?" Or, the question might be summarilly dismissed. Or, you may even be considered a likely candidate for psychological evaluation. Don't be deterred. You are entitled to the most serious consideration of your "question", especially if you have been under the care of a physician who has not been able to tell you what is causing your health problems. A subsequent chapter deals with what you can do to get an intelligent answer.

Many of the scientific papers investigating the mercury phenomenon have determined that some of the signs and symptoms associated with mercury exposure will ameliorate or disappear if the source of exposure is eliminated. This is possible if the cells of the impaired organs or function have not been damaged irreparably. It is accomplished simply by removing the source, and/or administering drugs or nutrients that tend to normalize function by binding with the mercury and removing it from the body via the urine or feces.

The key phrase in the above statement and in many of the scientific studies that have been done is "irreparable cell damage". Unfortunately, we are talking about very subtle and insidious cell damage that in most instances was never even looked for, or determined, because the studies or experiments were only attempting to determine one specific fact. The experiment protocols were simply not designed to detect possible cell damage in some other organ or system of the body.

As a result, many of our leading authorities in medicine and science tend to minimize the potential toxic effects of mercury except in those instances where there has been intoxication from known exposure. The operative words in that statement are INTOXICATION and KNOWN EXPOSURE. Micromercurialism I am afraid, never enters the picture.

This could be truly unfortunate for the millions of us who may be accumulating mercury in our bodies attributable to microdoses emanating from dental amalgam. The diagnosis, at best, is difficult and will be impossible if the health care provider you are seeing doesn't believe micromercurialism exists to begin with. How can you diagnose something if you don't believe it exists? Under that situation, the diagnostician is trying to tie your symptomatology to one of the diseases and/or conditions already defined and contained in the medical literature.

REFERENCES

1. Goodman and Gillman's. The Pharmacological Basis of Therapeutics. 6th Edition, 1980. Macmillan Publishing Co., Inc., New York.

2. Dorland's Illustrated Medical Dictionary. 25th Edition, 1974. W. B. Saunders Co., Philadelphia.

3. Report of an International Committee: Maximum allowable concentrations of mercury compounds. (MAC Values). Archives of Environmental Health, Vol. 19: pages 891–905, 1969.

4. Criteria for a recommended standard: Occupational Exposure to Inorganic Mercury. U.S. Department of Health, Education, and Welfare. Public Health Service. National Institute for Occupational Safety and Health, 1973.

4. Schafer, et al. A Textbook of Oral Pathology. 1974. W. B. Saunders Co., Philadelphia.

5. Trakhtenberg, I. M., Chronic Effects of Mercury on Organisms. U.S. Department of Health, Education, and Welfare. Publication Number (NIH) 74–473, 1974.

6. Gerstner, H. B., and Huff, J. E. Clinical Toxicology of Mercury. Journal of Toxicology and Environmental Health, Vol. 2, issue 3: pages 491–526, 1977.

7. Elhassani, S. B., The Many Faces of Methylmercury Poisoning. Journal of Toxicology: Clinical Toxicology, Vol. 19 issue 8, pages 875–906, 1982–1983.

8. Chang, L. W., Mercury In: Experimental and Clinical Neurotoxicology. Williams and Wilkins, 1980.

9. Mantyla, D. G., and Wright, O. D., Mercury Toxicity in The Dental Office: A Neglected Problem. Journal American Dental Association, Vol. 92, pages 1189–1194, 1976.

CHAPTER 9

ANECDOTES

Some of the dentists practicing mercury-free dentistry have been kind enough to provide me with some anecdotes or case histories. These all involve real, live people and are not figments of my imagination, the dentists', or the patients'. All of the case histories reflect documentation contained in either the dental records or the patient health history forms of the individuals concerned. Some I have personally interviewed. No names or locations have been included.

As stated in Chapter 2, anecdotal histories are normally not acceptable to the scientific community because they cannot be presented as statistical evidence and as a general rule are subject to human bias. It is a scientific fact that with some people, just the power of suggestion can cause the body to react in a favorable response. These are the individuals who after the administration of a "placebo" respond the same as if they had been administered medication. At least temporarily anyway.

From the researcher's standpoint, using or relating anecdotal evidence can be extremely frustrating. It immediately opens the door for criticism by his peers, be they dentist, physician or scientist. Those who criticize are also prone to disregard the hypothesis being developed through use of the anecdotes. For these individuals it is impossible for them to accept any evidence that is not derived from animal studies, or blind/double blind clinical trials. Therein lies a real tragedy for humanity. Mankind would be much better served if all those quick to denigrate would instead view the hypotheses and anecdotal histories objectively. If fully documented case histories are provided, together with a rational hypothesis, a more intelligent reaction would be to see if there was some scientific basis that could be proved, or disproved, through conventional research.

There is nothing wrong with healthy skepticism. However, it is slightly bizzare that a physician or group of physicians who may have diagnosed a major medical disease in a particular individual cannot accept as the truth, any amelioration in symptoms or an actual cure that doesn't result from the administration of a prescribed drug and/or surgery. I am not implying that all physicians feel that way. There are a great number of health care providers whose only concern is "that you were helped", regardless of the protocol.

There are a couple of serious cautions or warnings for those of you who feel any of the case histories sound exactly like your own situation. Don't assume anything and don't take any precipitous action without sound medical and dental advice. Chapter 10, outlines some courses of action that you as individuals can take. Read it carefully and proceed cautiously.

CASE 1

The individual is a white male who at the time of treatment was 61 years old. He is an engineer who had been exposed to mercury containing instruments most of his working life, ie., manometers, thermometers, etc., and also frequently had elemental mercury stored in his home.

He had previously been the patient of another dentist who did not believe anything about the potential toxicity of mercury from dental amalgam. Wanting to explore the problem further, he sought out his present dentist (who practices mercury-free dentistry) to get an evaluation as to whether mercury could possibly be involved in any of his varied health problems.

On November 11, 1983 he had his first appointment with the new dentist. The examination revealed that the patient had 6 amalgam surfaces (2 upper right and 4 upper left). He also had a 4 unit nickle/porcelain bridge on the lower left and a 3 unit nickle/porcelain bridge on the lower right. A complete medical history was taken and he was then evaluated for possible mercury toxicity/hypersensitivity. His diagnosis was possible mercury intoxication and the dentist recommended removal and replacement of the amalgam fillings with a composite. It was also recommended that the nickle bridges be replaced because of their potential carcinogenicity.

The patient's health history taken at the time of the initial visit revealed the following:

First amalgam fillings installed in 1943. Suffered incident of convulsions shortly thereafter. Also developed an allergic reaction to scallops shortly after placement of the fillings.

In 1945, while overseas with the armed forces, had 21 amalgam filling surfaces installed. Developed eczema right after the dental work was completed and was hospitalized for six months during which time he almost had one of his legs amputated because of the severity of the eczema.

In 1960, a gold bridge was installed on the upper right. He was hospitalized 1–2 months later with nausea and vomiting. He was diagnosed as having an ulcer, but did not respond to treatment. His immune system was found to be depressed and he was given antibiotics by IV.

During 1980–1981, patient was hospitalized 7 times. Diagnosed as having an inflamed pancreas that should be removed. Patient refused surgery. Was also diagnosed as having some deterioration of the right kidney, gall bladder, and liver.

Patient has had: continuous ear infections for 34 years; chronic headaches that would start in the occipital region, all of his adult life; for the past 15 years joint pains especially in his wrists and knees; abdominal pains for 30 years; paresthesia in his feet the last three years; tremors in his right arm and left leg; occasional uncontrollable hiccups; occasional chest pains and constipation; occasional cardiac bradycardia and missed beats; loss of visual accommodation; farsighted in the early 1960's. Patient says he is irritable, experiences anxiety, is unable to concentrate and feels he has had a decrease in memory, has suffered a loss of libido, is more introverted (shy), and has had an erythemetous rash, with itching and burning, especially on his legs, sternum and right facial cheek.

No depression, no fits of anger or loss of self control, no nightmares, and hearing is O.K.

Patient was referred to an M.D. for a coordinated protocol on Jan 11, 1984. On Feb 6, 1984, M.D. advised dentist that patient had recovered from a bleeding ulcer and that he would administer Vitamin C by IV the morning of his first dental appointment which was then scheduled for March 7, 1984.

March 7, 1984: 6 amalgam surfaces replaced with composite. (2 upper right and 4 upper left).

March 15, 1984: Removed 4 unit nickle/porcelain bridge from lower left. There were three amalgam surfaces under the bridge which were then replaced with composite.

March 22, 1984: Removed 3 unit nickle/porcelain bridge from lower right.

March 29, 1984: Delivered new porcelain fused to gold 4 unit bridge to lower left. Patient stated he is "feeling much better every week. Back pain is now totally gone".

April 5, 1984: Delivered new 3 unit porcelain fused to gold bridge to lower right. Patient stated "I am feeling great now". The patient also presented the dentist with a list of his symptoms and their chronology since he had started treatment. Changes in patient symptomatology started to occur on March 11, 1984: sneezing and headaches decreased but back pain and eczema increased. By March 27: back pain, neck stiffness, sneezing, coughing, eczema had all noticibly decreased. Headaches, dry throat and tooth aches had all ceased. By April 5, 1984: all symptoms had ceased with the exception of the eczema and earaches which had both decreased from moderate to light.

June 26, 1984: In a follow-up conversation with me the patient stated that the eczema and earaches had cleared entirely.

CASE 2

This 45 year-old Caucasian female was first seen by the dentist on April 8, 1983. She had requested the appointment after reading a newspaper article concerning the potential toxicity of dental amalgam. The dental examination included full mouth x-rays, evaluation of electrogalvanic potentials and a full consultation. The patient had a total of 30 amalgam surfaces in 11 teeth. Her health history and consultation revealed the following facts:

1980: Went to see her physician because of a numb feeling in her right nasal ala. Subsequent tests revealed liver abnormalities and neuritis. Patient was hospitalized for neurological evaluation, and other tests. The neurologist stated "right side not as good as left side. There was paresthesia on the entire right side of body". Bone scan, liver, spleen, skull, and barium enema were all normal. Resultant diagnosis was possibly "nerves".

Patient went to a chiropractor for an adjustment, who stated that she was slightly out of alignment, especially the atlas and occipitus. However, after adjustment, her body would not remain in alignment.

Patient went to visit another M.D. This physician stated he thought her problems might be related to mercury toxicity from her dental fillings because her throat was always red and burning (without any infection). Her nose was always stuffed; there was a pain in her right eye; a horrible taste in her mouth; joint pains in her right shoulder, elbow, knee and ankle. Patient also had consulted with a dermatologist concerning a skin rash which she frequently had all over her body. The dermatologist was unable to determine any cause for the rash.

The dental examination also revealed swollen lymph nodes under the right side of jaw and a click in the right TMJ. Dental diagnosis was possible mercury intoxication, with a recommendation that all dental amalgams be replaced with composites. The first appointment was scheduled for April 25, 1983.

4/25/83: Amalgams removed from 3 teeth on lower right (8 surfaces) and replaced with composite.

5/2/83: Patient stated "I can breathe a little better on my right side now. My hands and right side of my face are not as swollen. I started to notice improvement within hours of the initial amalgam replacement done on 4/25/83". Amalgams were removed from 3 teeth on the upper right (9 surfaces) and replaced with composites.

5/9/83: Patient's right nostril is completely clear now and

left nostril is opening slightly. Patient has noticed improvements 6 to 7 hours after removal of amalgams each time. Patient also has had green bowel movements after each session. Amalgams removed in 3 teeth (4 surfaces on lower left and 2 surfaces on upper right) and replaced with composites.

5/16/83: Remaining amalgams in 2 teeth (6 surfaces upper left) removed and replaced with composites. A total of 30 amalgam surfaces had been removed and replaced during the treatment plan.

2/17/84: Patient reported that she was doing great. There were no more breathing problems or swelling. Stated her physician wanted to know what she had done to improve so.

6/27/84: In a follow-up conversation with me, the patient stated that she was "much better all the way around". No more headaches, no metallic taste in her mouth, no more breathing problems or sore throat, and no more pressure build up behind her right eye.

CASE 3

Patient is a 48 year-old Caucasian female who was referred to this office by another dentist for determination of electrogalvanic potentials. The other dentist had administered a mercury patch test on August 26, 1983, which was positive but he did not want to remove the patient's amalgam fillings. On September 20, 1983, her first visit to the new dentist, there was still a red raised wheal at the site of the patch test area. The patient was examined and a health history taken that revealed the following information:

Patient had been diagnosed as having Lupus Erythemetosis two years previously. She had just gotten over a bad staph infection in her left eye for which she had received treatment at a medical clinic. Since then she had become allergic to codeine and sulfa drugs. Her previous dentist had advised her that she was also allergic to nickel. (Examination revealed a nickel-based porcelain to metal crown on the lower left 1st bicuspid).

Patient has had gastro-intestinal problems for the past 7–8 years; skin reactions for 15 years; far sightedness the last 6–7 years. No arthritis, no heart problems, no paresthesia, no tinnitus, and no headaches. Patient stated her skin rash had become worse 2 years ago, especially on neck, chest, stomach, and thighs.

Patient had 38 amalgam surfaces on 12 teeth. Dental diagnosis was possible mercury intoxication with a recommendation that all amalgam fillings be replaced with composites. First appointment was scheduled for November 2, 1983.

11/2/83: Area of mercury patch test still red and had a raised wheal. Amalgam fillings were removed from upper left 2nd molar (4 surfaces) and replaced with composite.

11/9/83: Patient reported she felt headachy after last appointment and the following day. Also had pain in lower right back the day following last appointment. Amalgam fillings were removed from 3 teeth on upper left (10 surfaces) and replaced with composites.

11/15/83: Amalgam fillings were removed from 3 teeth on lower left (9 surfaces) and replaced with composites.

11/30/83: Patient stated she has had intermittent dull headaches since last appointment but that they were beginning to ease. She also had a Lupus rash breakout on the medial and dorsal left ankle and medial left flank. Amalgam fillings removed from lower right (10 surfaces) and replaced with composites. Patient was feeling weak and nauseous after procedure. Blood pressure was 132/80.

12/7/83: Amalgam fillings removed on upper and lower right (9 surfaces) and replaced with composites.

1/11/84: Patient's Lupus Erythemous symptoms much improved. No more skin rashes. Eyesight seems better and eyes are less sensitive and not red. Removed crown on lower left 1st bicuspid and placed temporary composite full crown.

1/17/84: Patient reported eyes were red and irritated for 3 days after crown was removed. Physical condition much improved. No more skin rashes. Mouth less and less sensitive every day.

6/27/84: I called the patient to confirm the information contained in the dental records. The patient stated that her diagnosed Lupus condition had manifested itself primarily as skin rashes and that since replacement of her amalgam fillings she had been symptom free. She also stated that her eyes, which had always been bloodshot and for which she continually had to use eye drops, were no longer red. More importantly she said that the pressure build-up behind her eyes had disappeared.

CASE 4

Patient is a 37 year-old Caucasian male who was first seen on April 2, 1983. In October 1966, while on military service, patient had 4 small pit amalgam fillings placed. These were his first and only fillings. Patient's health history revealed the following:

October 1967: Hospitalized for severe malaise, lack of muscular control, could not walk. Base military hospital could not determine cause. Was sent to Chelsea Navy Hospital in Boston for further evaluation. A specific diagnosis could not be made but Multiple Sclerosis was suspected. Patient was discharged from military service. During the 1966–1967 period patient began wearing glasses, to correct for a myopic (near sighted) condition.

August 11, 1982: Hospitalized as a result of a heart attack. Suffered two more heart attacks during the next two weeks while still in the hospital. One week after 1st heart attack patient had kidney failure and was on dialysis for 72 days (as a result of all his health problems, he also lost his job). Patient had suffered pain in all major joints of body for 1 year prior to heart attack which became worse after his heart attacks. Also had chronic headaches for 4 months prior to heart attacks and had noticed diminished hearing during the year prior to his initial heart attack. Patient had been experiencing light-headedness and dizziness for 3–4 years prior to heart attacks and had also noticed a loss of short term memory during this same period.

While hospitalized for his heart attack, patient was diagnosed as being diabetic, although he had no previous history of diabetes. Had pancreatitis 1 month after heart attack, and also had his spleen removed at that time. Attending physician stated that patient's liver looked bad (patient states he was virtually a teatotaller and had no previous history of liver problems).

Patient had brought with him to his first appointment xrays from previous dentist. An electrogalvanic evaluation was done, and after consultation with patient, treatment plan for removal and replacement of amalgams was agreed to. At this time the patient's vital signs were: pulse 66, temperature 98.0, blood pressure, left arm 120/80, right arm 120/80. First appointment scheduled for April 13, 1983.

April 13, 1983: Vital signs prior to performing any dental work: pulse 78, temperature 97, blood pressure 118/80. Two small pit amalgam fillings on the upper right were removed and replaced with composite fillings. Vital signs 15 minutes after completion of dental work: pulse 72, temperature 98.6, blood pressure 120/84.

April 15, 1983: 2nd appointment. Patient stated his joint pains had totally cleared up for the first time since leaving the Navy and that he felt "good and stronger". Vital signs prior to dental work: pulse 68, temperature 98.0, blood pressure 120/74. Two small pit amalgam fillings on the upper left and lower right were removed and replaced with composite fillings. Vital signs 15 minutes after completion of dental work: pulse 68, temperature 98.0, blood pressure 120/80.

5/23/83: Patient called to say he was "doing great", no joint pains and feels better all around. Worked in the yard the first time in 7 years.

Patient has subsequently regained employment.

6/27/84: In a conversation with the patient he stated that replacement of his amalgam fillings had helped clear all of the problems he had previously reported.

CASE 5

Patient is a 47 year-old Caucasian female who called for the appointment after hearing a local radio talk show discussing the possibility of mercury toxicity from dental amalgam fillings.

Patient's health history revealed the following:

Bilateral mastectomy with mammoplasty due to fibrocystic nonmalignant lumps were performed in 1976. Three months later a hysterectomy was done to stop excessive bleeding.

Patient suffers with insomnia and cannot sleep more than one hour at a time; gets frequent headaches which start at back of neck; fatigues easily; has coordination difficulties; vision difficulties at times and chronic eye inflammation; has edema and is

constantly thirsty; chest pains; abdominal pain; generalized ar-
thritic condition not relieved by aspirin; is depressed with occasional thoughts of suicide; has throat constrictions. Patient also
stated she gets excrutiating pain throughout body which triggers
spasms in her jaw, feels like she will convulse. The pain and jaw
spasms started immediately after new braces were put on by her
orthodontist.

Patient was given a mercury patch test. Vital signs prior to
patch test were: pulse 78, temperature 99.0, blood pressure
102/70. One hour after patch was applied vital signs were: pulse
70, temperature 90, blood pressure 115/72. Patient got tingly,
prickly sensation in mouth. Patch was removed and test terminated because of reactions. Diagnosis was a positive reaction to
the mercury patch test.

Patient had 38 amalgam surfaces in 16 teeth. A treatment
plan was discussed and agreed to and the first appoinment was
scheduled for July 1, 1983.

7/1/83: Amalgams removed from three teeth on lower left (8
surfaces) and replaced with composite fillings.

7/4/83: Patient was called to see how she was doing. Patient
stated "best I've felt in 10 years, slept four hours straight.
Cleaned the house and still had energy".

7/5/83: Patient called at 4:15 P.M. and stated she was having
symptoms of diarrhea, a sensation of bladder or kidney infection
starting, and was passing blood in urine. She was told to contact
her physician immediately and that her appointment for 7/6/83
would be cancelled.

7/6/83: Patient called at 8:15 A.M. and stated she was doing
100% better. Her appointment was rescheduled for 7/9/83.

7/9/83: Amalgams removed from four teeth on lower right
(11 surfaces) and replaced with composite fillings.

7/13/83: Dentist consulted with the orthodontist and both
agreed patient would be better off with braces removed. Amalgams removed from four teeth upper left (6 surfaces) and replaced with composite fillings.

7/16/83: Remaining amalgams removed from five teeth on
upper right (13 surfaces) and replaced with composite fillings.

6/27/83: I called patient to confirm information reflected on
the dental records. During the course of the conversation patient

brought out the fact that she had also been diagnosed as having Multiple Sclerosis and that this condition was now cleared up. She attributed the resolution of the MS to the removal and replacement of the amalgam fillings and to subsequent treatment received from a holistic physician. During the latter treatment an allergy to wheat was diagnosed and she has carefully avoided wheat to the best of her ability.

CASE 6

he patient is a 58 year-old Oriental female who was first seen on June 24, 1983. Consultation and patient health history revealed the following information:

Patient stated she was diagnosed as having rheumatoid arthritis in 1957 approximately two years after having all her amalgam fillings removed and replaced with new amalgam fillings. Her dentist in Maryland advised her to have this done because her old fillings were deteriorating and there was decay under some of the fillings. Patient moved to Florida in 1958 and had taken aspirin for her arthritis condition for over 20 years. Patient had undergone gold treatments for her arthritis but had developed a rash. She had also had DMSO treatments which seemed to help her arthritis. Patient has a raw burning feeling in mouth and throat and has suffered some loss of hearing. Patient had knot on back of right hand and stated she had similar knots all over her body. Also stated she was very allergic to poison ivy.

Patient was given a mercury patch test. Vital signs prior to test were: pulse 88, temperature 98.6, blood pressure 104/66. Vital signs one hour after patch was applied: pulse 90, temperature 99, blood pressure 116/78. Patch test was terminated with a diagnosis of positive reaction to mercury.

Patient had 26 amalgam surfaces in 14 teeth. Patient also had one gold inlay. A treatment plan was discussed and agreed to with the first appointment scheduled for July 13, 1983.

7/13/83: Amalgams removed from three teeth on lower left (7 surfaces) and replaced with composite fillings. Removed gold inlay from lower left 1st bicuspid. There was an amalgam filling under the gold and the tooth had necrotic (dead) pulp. Placed temporary crown and recommended that root canal therapy be performed.

7/20/83: Amalgams removed from two teeth on lower right (7 surfaces) and replaced with composite fillings.

8/5/83: Amalgams removed from two teeth on upper right (4 surfaces) and replaced with composite fillings.

8/17/83: Amalgams removed from four teeth on upper left (8 surfaces) and replaced with composite fillings.

10/3/83: Patient called and stated she is getting better very slowly. Joints are not quite as sore.

11/4/83: Patient called and stated she is gradually getting better.

11/9/83: Impression taken for replacement crown.

11/29/83: Patient stated swelling in hands and joints has gone down considerably and that she has increased gripping strength in both hands. Delivered porcelain fused to gold full crown with cast gold core.

6/27/84: I called the patient to see what her physical condition was 7 months after treatment had been completed. The patient stated that her arthritis condition had ameliorated quite a bit but that she still had a lot of pain. She also stated that she had not been able to follow the detoxification program outlined by her dentist to reduce her total mercury body burden. She said her stomach was so sensitive from having taken aspirin for so many years that she couldn't take any vitamin C. As a result she could not take the cysteine either. This fact has been brought to the attention of her dentist who will try to work up a protocol that she can follow.

In closing this chapter on anecdotal experiences I would like to quote two additional case histories. These will be quoted in their entirety exactly as published. Please take special note of the dates of these articles as they serve to reinforce the fact that the problem is certainly not new.

This case was published in Dental Cosmos, Vol. XIII, 1871, pages 637–638.

MISCELLANY
ABSTRACTS AND SELECTIONS
By J. W. WHITE

Dental Times

Dr. Elihum R. Pettit gives a case in practice, showing the "Injurious Effects of Amalgam."

"On October 1st, 1868, I inserted a large amalgam filling in the second inferior left molar, mesial and grinding surfaces. On the 8th of the same month the patient, Mrs. P. ate two or three fried oysters and almost immediately afterward became very sick at the stomach—without vomiting, however, but with a rash breaking out upon her face and neck, with itching, and oedema of the face and eyelids. But the next day she was quite well, except that the rash had not entirely disappeared. About a month afterward, again partaking of oysters, the same symptoms returned, with coldness of the extremities, to such a degree as to become alarming. Attributing these symptoms to the oysters, she abstained from them entirely.

"On the 17th of May, 1870, I applied the arsenical paste to the pulp of the right inferior second molar tooth of the same patient, in the usual manner. About an hour later, after the lady had returned to her home, the symptoms above mentioned reappeared. She returned the next day, when I cleaned out the cavity and removed the pulp. The rash had then partially disappeared. On the succeeding day, the 19th, when she returned to have the tooth filled she complained of all her teeth being sore, and some of them slightly loose, but especially those on the right side of the mouth and in the immediate neighborhood of the tooth to the pulp of which the paste had been applied. The rash had also returned in a greater degree than before. I am quite confident that the patient could not have swallowed any of the paste, although the cavity was on the proximal surface and the tooth was properly protected by napkins, so that these effects must have been produced entirely by the absorption of the arsenious acid through the pulp. The patient left the city the same day, the 19th, and while absent the same symptoms were produced by fish and radishes.

"The similarity of these symptoms with those produced

long before by the oyster point to the same cause for both, as there had previously been no idiosyncrasy in regard to any article of food. Upon careful examination no cause could be discovered why such effects should be produced, when, to test the matter, I removed the amalgam filling, supposing that the mercury might have produced and kept up such a state of irritability in the system that articles of food, which might have even a slight tendency to disagree with her, even if not sufficient to be noticed, might produce such alarming results. Since that time (May, 1870), there has been no return of the symptoms, although she has partaken freely of oysters and such other food as before disagreed with her, thus proving these effects to have been caused by the mercury.

"Although such cases are rare, they are sufficiently frequent to cause us to be on our guard against them, while they should lead us to discard from our practice, wherever it is possible to do so, a substance so insidiously deleterious in its effects. They should lead us also to remove all amalgam from the teeth of any of our patients, who may have been suffering from ill health from any obscure or uncertain cause, which will not yield to the ordinary remedies; while those who are in the habit of inserting such fillings generally, making gold the exception, incur a responsibility which few, who are aware of such cases, would care to assume."

The second article appeared in the Periscope section of The Dental Cosmos, Vol. XVI, 1874, pages 213–214.

"POISONING FROM CORROSIVE SUBLIMATE GENERATED IN THE MOUTH FROM AMALGAM PLUGS IN THE TEETH—Having been invited by an eminent gentleman of the medical profession to attend a convention of the State Medical Society to submit to its consideration a matter of vital importance to the human family, and being unable to comply with the invitation, I have written this article to lay the matter before the medical profession and ask its cooperation.

The matter which I wished to bring to the notice of the profession is the poisoning of thousands of people all over the world from corrosive sublimate generated in the mouth from amalgam plugs in the teeth. Neither Asiatic cholera, nor smallpox, nor any malarious disease is doing half the mischief in the

world that is being done by this poisoning. Every medical man of
any considerable practice has undoubtedly had numerous cases
of it, but never knew what it was. The symptoms are so numerous and varied in different cases that it would be impossible to
give them all in this short article, but I will say that a person is
liable to be treated for dyspepsia, neuralgia, paralysis, consumption, and numerous throat-diseases. The patient gradually
wastes away as if going into a decline, and no medicine will
afford any relief. In many cases the difficulty steals on so gently
as not to excite the least alarm, and continues very gradually for
a number of years till the patient becomes a total wreck; while in
others the attack comes on violently, and the friends and attending physician think the patient is dying; but he will again rally,
and again be prostrated.

There is such a resemblance in the symptoms to nearly all
the diseases to which human flesh is heir that the physician is led
to treat the patient for some disease which seems to be a very
clear case, but his patient gets worse. In more than twenty cases
that I have had, nearly all had been pronounced by some physician as having consumption. In nearly all the cases there are at
times a very bad cough, eyes sunken, and haggard expression
and deep blue or dark color under the eyes, invariably a metallic
taste in the mouth, water flowing from the mouth in the night
while asleep so as to wet the pillow, and in most cases extreme
prostration.

I have not time now to detail the manner in which the corrosive sublimate is formed in the mouth, further than to say that
the quicksilver in the plugs is driven off by the heat of the mouth
in very minute particles, and, combining with the chlorine in the
fluids of the mouth, or any saline substance, such as our food,
passes into the stomach, and produces slow poisoning. If the
State Medical Society will appoint a committee to visit this
place, I will show them several cases that will place the matter
beyond controversy.

There are some twelve thousand dentists in the United
States doing a wholesale business at this poisoning, and I ask the
cooperation of the State Medical Society, as guardians of the
public health, to assist in getting an act of Congress passed making it a penitentiary offense to place any poisonous substance in

teeth that will injure the people.—J. Payne, D.D.S., in Chicago Medical Journal.''

Sound familiar? Science has progressed light years since that article appeared in 1874 but has anything changed? The recommendations made by Dr. Payne in 1874 are just as valid today as they were then. Professionals talking to professionals will not change the situation. The only way the problem will ever be solved is for the general public, the recipients of mercury amalgam fillings, to raise their voices to a level that Congress and the Establishment can recognize. Which, unfortunately in this day and age of vested interests, has to be pretty loud.

Chapter 10 provides a list of actions you can take to help bring an end to this 150 year old war.

CHAPTER 10

WHAT CAN I DO?

The first thing that you must do, is make an individual and personal decision about what you have read. If you do not believe that the mercury in dental amalgam or dissimilar metals in the mouth represent a potentially serious health hazard, then merely count the time expended reading this book as "contributing to your total store of interesting facts" and turn your attention to other things.

If, on the other hand, you reach a conclusion that there appears to be some basis to the statements that dissimilar metals can create electrical havoc in your body and that mercury and other metals escaping from dental amalgam and entering your body constitute potentially serious threats to human health then, be assured, there are a whole range of actions that you can take.

On the personal level, there are three categories or levels of action that you can take:

1. The first category only requires stationery, a writing implement and suitable postage. This involves the simple act of requesting that your elected representatives, and the appropriate agencies of the federal government resolve the questions. Suitable research projects and protocols must be established and funded to answer the questions scientifically.

A. Write to your Senator and Congressman expressing your

concerns and request that they provide you with an answer as to what the U.S. Government is going to do to:

(1) Determine the safety of mercury amalgam dental filling materials. Also request that you be provided with an explanation why the government agencies charged with public health and safety have allowed private associations and industry to make the final judgements on the issues involved.

(2) Provide an acceptable rationale to explain why there hasn't been any composite material approved for posterior use when research data has shown some are equally as good if not better than amalgam.

(3) Explain why representatives of private organizations are permanently in place at the National Bureau of Standards and can impose parochial interests to influence the type of research being done on dental materials.

(4) Explain how The American Dental Association and insurance companies can be the deciding factor on what dental filling material the patient will receive and that the dentist can use. The cost of health care today makes it extremely difficult for the average patient to obtain needed service without insurance payment.

B. Write to Dr. James B. Wyngaarden, Director, National Institutes of Health, 14 North Drive, Bethesda Maryland, 20814:

Request that you be provided with scientific proof supporting statements made by the various divisions under his control and the ADA that the small amount of mercury escaping from dental amalgams and being absorbed by the body causes no pathological damage and does not constitute a health hazard.

Ask how is it possible that in all the billions of dollars expended on research projects, nobody has ever demanded that toxicological research on heavy metals include dental amalgam as a source.

C. Write to the Honorable Margaret M. Heckler, Secretary, Health and Human Services, 200 Independence Ave. S.W., Washington D.C., 20201, and request an explanation as to why the Food and Drug Administration has not seen fit to subject the use of mercury amalgam dental material to the same intensive review that all other poisonous substances dispensed as drugs are and have been.

You should also request an answer as to why all future health statistics and epidemiological studies of the U.S. population cannot be subdivided into two groups, those with amalgam fillings and those without.

2. If you have been under a physician's care for any of the diseases or syndrome type health conditions (collection of symptoms) for which there is no established etiology or cause and you have mercury amalgam fillings in your mouth then you should take the following actions.

Return to your physician and discuss with him the possibility that mercury hypersensitivity or intoxication may be involved. If he or she doesn't think much of the idea, then start calling other physicians until you find one who has an open mind, has knowledge on the subjects of mercury toxicity and/or hypersensitivity, and is willing to work with you to try and find an answer.

An allergist can determine whether you are hypersensitive to mercury, or some of the other metals contained in the amalgam.

Blood tests can determine the mercury content of the blood. Unfortunately, the results provide very inconclusive correlations to tissue toxicity. Perhaps more importantly, White Blood Cell and T Cell and B Cell lymphocyte counts can provide very important clues. If the latter tests show decreased counts and there are no other obvious medical conditions that can be attributed to the results, then recent research that has shown depression of lymphocyte counts by mercury, should suggest to your physician that serious consideration be given to the possibility that amalgam fillings may be the causative factor.

Your physician can prescribe oral detoxification using some of the drugs that have been demonstrated to be effective in binding mercury. Urinalysis while undergoing this type of treatment will indicate whether you are excreting increased amounts of mercury in your urine. This should provide an indication that you are decreasing your total body burden of mercury. There may also be an amelioration of symptoms which would be an additional factor implicating mercury.

If your particular philosophy of life does not encompass the taking of drugs, the detoxification of mercury can also be accomplished using certain natural substances. Scientific research has shown that the amino acid Cysteine (not cystine) has a specific affinity for mercury and will bind with it permitting excretion of the mercury from your body. (Sprince Etal, Fed. Proc. Vol 33, no. 3, Part 1 March 1974) There is a relationship between Vitamin C and Cysteine that must be maintained if it is to be effective. The ratio of C to Cysteine is 3 to 1. For example, if you take 500 milligrams of Cysteine, you must take 1500 milligrams of vitamin C.*

Afterwards, if there is some correlation to mercury indicated by the tests, then your physician in all probability will recommend that you see your dentist about having your amalgam fillings removed and replaced with one of the new composite materials or with gold.

3. Or, you may elect to first discuss the problem with your dentist. Unfortunately at this point, as with most physicians, too many of them are not conversant with all the scientific literature on dental amalgam's potential toxicity. They are only aware of the position that has been taken by the ADA that only a handful of people are hypersensitive to mercury.

If your dentist starts treating you as a child, explaining that amalgam is perfectly safe and has been used for 150 years, thank him for the lesson in history and go find yourself another dentist. As with the criteria for finding a physician, find a dentist who has an open mind, but more importantly, find one who has taken the time and effort to inform himself or herself on the subject and knows the correct procedures and has the equipment and materials required.

Serious efforts are underway to compile national lists of dentists who practice mercury-free dentistry and who are conversant with all the latest procedures and protocols. Some of the organizations or individuals compiling such lists are:

Toxic Testing Inc., Suite 232
303 E. Altamonte Drive
Altamonte Springs, Florida 32701

Their nationwide Toll-Free phone number is 1-800-327-8885.

*Sprince Etal Fed. Proc. Vol. 33, No. 3 Part 1 March 1974 and Oeriv Bochitu, Journal of Gerontology, Vol. 20 P. 417, 1965

Dr. Hal Huggins, P.O. Box 2589, Colorado Springs, CO 80906.
Dr. Jerry Mittelman, 263 West End Ave., #21, New York, N.Y.
10023
Dr. Roy Kupsinal, P.O. Box 550, Oviedo, FL 32765
Bio-Probe, Inc. 4401 Real Ct., Orlando FL 32808

There are several different ways available to you and your
health care provider to determine whether your mercury amalgam fillings and/or dissimilar metals are contributing to your
total body burden of mercury and/or creating potentially dangerous levels of electrogalvanic action in your mouth:

Toxic Testing, Inc. offers a Pre-Screen Evaluation Test.
This is a questionnaire type screening that is designed to tell you
whether you may be prone to mercury hypersensitivity and
whether you should pursue the question further with your dentist. Some dentists are using the pre-screen evaluation routinely.
If your dentist has an open mind and wants to work with you,
ask him to get the test, or you contact Toxic Testing Inc. directly. There is a nominal charge for this service.

Some dental offices are equipped to provide the following
services:

Jerome or Bachrach Mercury Vapor Analyzer evaluations.
With these instruments the dentist can perform a simple non-
invasive test to determine how much mercury vapor is being
released from your amalgam fillings. Readings are taken in your
mouth before and after chewing gum for 5 or 10 minutes. High
readings after chewing would tend to confirm that anytime you
are chewing, you are inhaling and ingesting mercury vapor and/
or abraded particles and contributing to your total body burden
of mercury.

Evaluations by Electrodentogram or Amalgameter. These
are instruments that are capable of determining the electrical
potentials or currents being generated by dissimilar metals in the
mouth. High readings could possibly be involved in a number of
health problems from pain, headaches or temperomandibular
joint (TMJ) dysfunction in addition to causing increased corrosion and increased release of mercury from the amalgam fillings.

Evaluation by mercury patch testing. This is a simple test
for skin and systemic reaction to a very dilute solution of mercuric chloride that is placed on a patch and taped to the arm.

There is some controversy concerning the patch test at this time. The ADA has stated that it is possible to sensitize some individuals to mercury simply by giving them the patch test and they have recommended to their members that only qualified allergists should perform the test. Regardless of who might administer the patch test, there are some prohibitions on giving the test to the following individuals: Pregnant women, diagnosed cases of Systemic Lupus Erythematosis, Multiple Sclerosis, Leukemia, Hodgkins disease, cardiovascular disease, mental illness (especially manic depression), Acrodynia, and MLNS (Kawasaki's disease). SPECIAL NOTE—if you have made up your mind to have your amalgam fillings replaced, do not take the mercury patch test.

There are also a couple of things you can do in the way of self-evaluation. First is taking your oral temperature. There is evidence in the scientific literature indicating that mercury can cause sub-normal temperatures. If your oral temperature, checked at the same time on successive days, consistently reads below 98.6 degrees Farenheit, it could be an indication that total mercury body burden may be involved.

One last thing you can do is to play detective on yourself. Take a sheet of paper and start jotting down the approximate dates of when your chronic or consistent symptoms of health problems started appearing. For example, when you first started feeling extremely tired or fatigued all the time, or when you first started having recurrent headaches, or when did you first start having severe acne, or when did you first notice that metallic taste in your mouth, etc. etc. In this regard, you might consult the Chapter 8 listing of symptoms and pick out the problems you have and when they started.

Next, to the best of your knowledge, jot down the dates when you first had any dental restoration type work done, and all subsequent dates when additional work was done. Remember now, we are also talking about dissimilar metals and this would include the installation of any metal in your mouth, including orthodontic devices.

Lastly, line up the two sets of dates and see if there is any relationship between when you first experienced the symptoms and when you had the dental work done. You might turn up some astonishing correlations.

Bear in mind that there is no one test that will tell you categorically that amalgams and/or electrogalvanic potentials are the cause of your problems. In many cases it will be a subjective judgement similar to concluding "that where there's smoke, there could be fire".

You personally have to be the ultimate judge of how much proof you need in order to make up your own mind that the health problems you have been experiencing may be related to your amalgam fillings or dissimilar metals in your mouth. If you decide that there is a very probable relationship and you want to proceed with removal of the metals and replacement with the newer composites, exercise caution. A great number of dentists are still not familiar with the new composite materials used for posterior restorations or the proper techniques for their correct installation.

Don't be bashful. Ask your dentist which brands of composites he has been using and how long he has been using them and whether the manufacturer has stated that the material is acceptable for posterior use. Have him explain exactly what his treatment plan is and what you can expect to happen.

In most instances, the removal of the amalgam fillings will temporarily increase your body burden of mercury and may cause an exacerbation of your symptoms. Your dentist should be completely familiar with the nutritional support/detoxification protocol that you should be on concurrently with any removal of amalgams, and the length of time you should remain on such protocols. In most instances where a great number of amalgam surfaces are involved, your dentist should schedule you for multiple appointments. You should be on a nutritional support/detoxification program for the entire period and for 30 days after removal of the last amalgam.

This is no panacea. With a great number of individuals, you may begin to experience relief or amelioration of symptomatology within the first week after some of the amalgams have been replaced. Others may not experience any changes until all of the amalgams have been replaced and their body has had sufficient time to excrete and reduce the total body burden of mercury. This can be anywhere from one week to six months after the last amalgam has been replaced.

Finally, there are those of us who may not experience a relief or changes in symptomatology. Remember, each of us has a specific biochemical individuality that will ultimately determine how we respond. No matter what the outcome, you will have done one thing that is irrefutable. You will have eliminated a potential source of continual contamination to your body systems and in those individuals where dissimilar metals can be totally eliminated, you will have removed the source for the generation of any potentially harmful electrical potentials.

For those of you who have had their amalgams or dissimilar metals replaced I would very much like to hear the results. Please provide as much detail as you can in your case history. Include the name, address, and phone number of your dentist or physician (if he was involved).

I intend to keep compiling anecdotal evidence until the entire question concerning the continued use of amalgam fillings has been satisfactorily resolved. You may write to me at the following address:

Sam Ziff
4401 Real Ct.,
Orlando FL 32808.

AURORA PRESS

Barbara Somerfield is pleased to announce the birth of Aurora Press, a company devoted to publishing books that catalyze personal growth, balance and transformation.

Aurora Press will provide a publishing vehicle for an innovative synthesis of ancient wisdom with twentieth century resources.

Aurora books specialize in astrology, tarot, the healing arts, color therapy, acupuncture, and the emerging global consciousness.

THE DANE RUDHYAR SERIES

We are particularly proud to publish the books of Dane Rudhyar, internationally recognized astrologer, composer, poet, artist and philosopher who initiated the concept of a humanistic and transpersonal approach to life.

THE PLANETARIZATION OF CONSCIOUSNESS

The Planetarization of Consciousness is Rudhyar's major philosophical work, the concentrated outcome of a lifetime of thinking concerning the most basic problems of human existence and the meaning of the radical social-cultural and psychological crisis mankind is experiencing.
Paper 320pp. $9.95

THE GALACTIC DIMENSION OF ASTROLOGY
The Sun is Also a Star
A deepened understanding of Uranus, Neptune and Pluto can guide us towards experiencing the galactic level of consciousness. The "challenge of galacticity" to humanistic astrology releases new perspectives when applied to individual horoscopes. His new interpretations of the trans-Saturnian planets provide a vehicle to transform how we use astrology in our daily lives, and for the evolving planet we live on.
Paper 224pp. $7.95

ASTROLOGICAL INSIGHTS INTO THE SPIRITUAL LIFE
Astrological Insights provides a penetrating, sensitive, poetic and visual insight into the 12 qualities required for the spiritual life, for Astrologers and non-astrologers alike. Using the astrological signs and houses, Rudhyar builds a framework for impregnating the seeker with an awareness of how to use basic life challenges, as a process through which an individual human being evolves. Twelve exquisite artistic renderings evoke the archetypal, intuitive level of each sign.
Paper 160pp. $7.95

AN ASTROLOGICAL TRYPTICH
In *Tryptich* Rudhyar extracts from traditional astrology a great wealth of psychological and spiritual meaning. New interpretations of the zodiacal signs, houses and planets shed light on the three basic phases of spiritual unfoldment. *Tryptich* is a book to read and reread! Each chapter stands by itself, yet as a part in a vast symphony of revealed values and inspired imagery.
Paper 320pp. $9.95

ASTROLOGICAL ASPECTS:
A Process Oriented Approach
with Leyla Rael Rudhyar
A cyclic and holistic approach to aspects including chapters on retrogradation, rectangular and triangular aspect patterns, seeing the horoscope intuitively as a whole, Yods, an explanation of the three types of every planetary aspect with examples and practical applications.
Paper 244pp. $9.95

PERSON CENTERED ASTROLOGY
Lucid and inspiring material on the purpose of Astrology in New Age guidance and the difference between an event-oriented approach and a person centered view. Illustrated with complete case studies, concrete examples of the holistic approach in action and practical technique.
Paper 385pp. $10.95

THE LUNATION PROCESS IN ASTROLOGICAL GUIDANCE
Leyla Rael Rudhyar
The only book available on the use of the Progressed Lunation Cycle as a tool in process oriented Life Interpretation. The technique, theory, and phases are explained in detail with several whole life case histories to illustrate the use of this valuable technique.
Paper 62pp. $3.95

AURORA PRESS

THE ELISABETH HAICH SERIES

Through books such as *Initiation*, Elisabeth Haich has become world famous for her profound understanding of the human soul. The Yoga schools she set up in Europe with Selvarajan Yesudian have become internationally renowned.

WISDOM OF THE TAROT

Wisdom of the Tarot relates the path of higher consciousness through the color, shape and symbolic forms on the 22 cards. Detailed study of a Tarot card may release instinctive awareness of each level towards the Light. When studied individually, a card may reveal the necessary steps to find one's essential path. Included are 5 color gold Tarot cards.

Paper 174pp. $12.50

SEXUAL ENERGY & YOGA

This book is to introduce the concept of transmuting the physical emotional psychic mental energy people normally disperse in sexual activity for the purpose of uniting their bodies in their higher Self or God.

Paper 160pp $6.95

THE EAR

Gateway to Balancing the Body
A Modern Guide to Ear Acupuncture
Mario Wexu, D. Ac.

This is the first complete modern textbook of ear acupuncture. Anatomical descriptions with detailed charts clearly illustrate how to locate and use over 300 ear points, both alone and in combination with body points, to treat and prevent illness. An excellent repertory listing 150 diseases facilitates an indepth understanding of this incredible and valuable healing art.

Cloth 203pp. $30.00

COLOR THERAPY

Dr. Reuben Amber

This comprehensive book enumerates the myriad ways we can consciously choose to use color to influence our body, mind, and soul to promote balanced health and well being. No other book includes as thorough a historical survey of Color Therapies along with specific applications of color in all facets of life.

Paper 207pp. $9.95

HOW COSMIC & ATMOSPHERIC ENERGIES INFLUENCE YOUR HEALTH

Dr. Michel Gauquelin

A unique exploration by psychologist and statistician Dr. Michel Gauquelin, of the tremendous influence of the cycle of the seasons, range of climates, cosmic clocks, Lunar Cycles, & Sunspots on the complex balance of mental and physical health.

Paper 224pp. $8.95

SELF HEALING, YOGA AND DESTINY

Designed to reconnect you with the Divine, the concepts within this book explain the attitudes necessary for the path back to one's Self. Based on many years personal experience, the author creates a vehicle to realize the essential source of Life, especially in relation to illness and self healing.

Paper 80pp. $4.95

THE DAY WITH YOGA

A different creative energy is at work on each day of the week. In this book Elisabeth Haich has carefully chosen and collected quotations which show us how we can attune to the cosmic vibrations of each day.

Paper 96pp. $3.95

CHART INTERPRETATION —

Astrology and Psychology
Doris Hebel

A compilation of articles on Chart Interpretation, covering Elements, aspects, hemisphere emphasis, retrogrades, stations, parental indicators, and case histories.

Paper 64pp. $5.

SYNASTRY

Understanding Human Relations
Through Astrology   *Ronald Davison*

This book contains the first comprehensive survey of the various techniques of horoscope comparison.

The author has discovered "The Relationship Horoscope," an entirely new way of charting in a single horoscope the relationship between two people. He also introduces new methods of determining the quality of that relationship.

Paper 352pp. $10.95

AWAKEN HEALING ENERGY THROUGH THE TAO

Mantak Chia

This unique book reveals the ancient Taoist secret of circulating internal energy through acupuncture meridians, for physical, psychological and spiritual health. Written in clear, easy to understand language and illustrated with many detailed diagrams that aid the development of a powerful energetic flow.

Paper 224pp. $10.95